Appreciating Practice in the Caring Professions

Refocusing Professional Development and Practitioner Research

Della Fish PhD, MA, MEd, BA Hons, Dip Ed

Consultant in Educational and Professional Development
Honorary Research Fellow, School of Education,
Exeter University

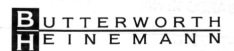

OXFORD   BOSTON   JOHANNESBURG   MELBOURNE   NEW DELHI   SINGAPORE

Butterworth-Heinemann
Linacre House, Jordan Hill, Oxford OX2 8DP
225 Wildwood Avenue, Woburn MA 01801-2041
A division of Reed Educational and Professional Publishing Ltd

℞ A member of the Reed Elsevier plc group

First published in 1998

British Library Cataloguing in Publication Data

A catalogue record for this book is available from the British Library

Library of Congress Cataloguing in Publication Data

A catalogue record for this book is available from the Library of
Congress

ISBN 0 7506 3001 9

Printed and bound in Great Britain by Biddles Ltd., Guildford and
Kings Lynn

PLANT A TREE
*British Trust for
Conservation Volunteers*
FOR EVERY TITLE THAT WE PUBLISH, BUTTERWORTH-HEINEMANN
WILL PAY FOR BTCV TO PLANT AND CARE FOR A TREE.

Contents

List of figures and tables

Acknowledgements

Formal thanks are due to the Musée des Beaux Arts de Belgique for supplying the photograph of *Paysage avec la chute d'Icare* by Pieter Bruegel, and Faber and Faber for permission to reproduce the poem by W. H. Auden from *Collected Shorter Poems* (1968). This book would never have been written without the generous support of many friends in the caring professions. Particularly I acknowledge with grateful thanks the influence and help of Colin Coles, Professor of Medical Education, Bournemouth University, whose special contributions are acknowledged in the text, and Sam Dawson, lately of Swansea University, who read an early draft and commented helpfully on material now in Part Two. Others who offered special help and encouragement are: Sarah Beeston, Head of Department of Rehabilitation Sciences, University of East London; Gill Brown, Head Occupational Therapist, Community Paediatrics, Redbridge Health Care Trust; Harrie Broekman, Education Advisor, IVLOS, Universitiet Utrecht; Ann Hopper, Honorary Research Fellow, Exeter University; Susan Ryan, Reader, Department of Rehabilitation Sciences, University of East London; Ken Shifrin, Dean of the College of Traditional Acupuncture, Leamington Spa; Sheila Twinn, Principal Lecturer in Nursing at the Chinese University of Hong Kong; and Jasmine Uddin, chair of the British Acupuncture Council.

I acknowledge with gratitude the help and support during the preparation of this publication from Susan Devlin, senior medical editor for Butterworth-Heinemann, and her editorial assistant, Helen Reece.

I am – as ever – grateful to Jean Douglas and Evelyn Usher who have borne the burden of extensive reading of early drafts and the correcting of later proofs with great fortitude and good will. Their support in all its forms has been invaluable.

Any opinions expressed are entirely mine and are in no way associated with any institution or official body for which I work.

Della Fish

Introduction

Mapping the territory: a brief overview of the argument

Intentions

The ideas behind the term 'professional artistry' offer a new way forward for practitioners in the caring professions who are beginning to recognize how overshadowed they have been by ideas and processes imposed from outside. Technical imperatives, proceduralization, scientific research and government policies have all told practitioners what they must do and how they must do it. But none of these actually helps us to *understand, explain or develop* our *own* practice. Such processes have ignored issues about why we work as we do. They change us, but only on the outside. As a result, we have altered our ways of working (to suit the ideas of others) but not refocused our thinking and seeing. Worse, we have not created and defended ways of working that are right for us as professionals.

The term 'professional artistry' has been around for several decades, but the details of what it involves, and its implications for practitioners seem never to have been fully worked out. The term is used throughout this book to indicate that a holistic view of practice is taken. This subsumes into a much broader picture of practice the skills which are a springboard for, but which are not the only characteristic of, successful practice. These skills, procedures and all other visible elements of practice (which are *all* that the technical rational view of practice is interested in) are here seen as only a small part of a professional's work in a practice setting. Professional artistry is concerned with these but also with the invisible aspects of practice, which though hidden are far more extensive than its visible elements. These include the practitioner's capacities, abilities, assumptions, theories, beliefs, values, and the moral dimensions of practice, including the practitioner's professional judgements.

Why does this view of professional practice matter to those of us who are at the heart of the daily work of the caring professions? What are the advantages, and further, what are the practical implications and obligations of recognizing and focusing on the artistry of practice? How can practitioner research do justice to professional artistry? How can the professional development of the artist practitioner be provided for? This book sets out to explore these matters. It seeks to open colleagues' eyes to the ways in which recognizing the artistry of professional practice can fundamentally change the agenda for, and processes of, practitioner research and professional development. This view puts practitioners at the heart of professional development and research rather than being the mere subjects and recipients of them, and makes the investigation of practice by practitioners its central activity.

The ideas and processes discussed here will enable practitioners at all stages in the profession – those who are students, those who are in the thick of daily professional practice, those who are taking time out to research their practice – to investigate in detail and learn from aspects of their work. Indeed, much of what is discussed here has *emerged from* practice – the practice of professionals who, during the normal course of their day-to-day work in a range of caring professions, have sought through systematic enquiry to understand their practice and its artistry (see Fish and Coles, 1998). Whilst being free standing, this book is also a sequel to Fish and Coles, 1998.

The audience

Throughout this book the term 'caring professions' is used to encompass all those professions in which the good of the client in terms of health, education and/or social matters is the foremost concern of the professional. The specific audience targeted is professional practitioners, practitioner teachers and student practitioners as well as managers, in all the health care professions whose work is related to Western medicine, and in education (school teaching and teacher education). Members of other professions, like those of social work and those offering alternative therapies based upon Traditional Chinese Medicine, should also find the principles and processes discussed here entirely relevant. Detailed references to their literature and practices are however unfortunately beyond the scope of this text.

The term 'appreciation'

At the very core of the kind of professional development discussed here is the term 'appreciation'. It flags a changed direction and a different intention for professional development and practitioner research from that shaped by traditional scientific approaches and bureaucratic concerns. The term comes from the Arts (where it is sometimes referred to as a 'critique', 'practical criticism' or a 'critical commentary') and it is concerned with recognizing in a sensitive and holistic way the qualities of practice – with recognizing and responding to a piece of practice seen as artistry – and with thinking critically about the values, traditions, beliefs and assumptions which underlie its surface. Its view of truth, proof, rigour and validity is different from that found within the study of science. But it is no less rigorous and disciplined. Its focus is a particular piece of practice but this – as is also necessary in critical appreciation in the Arts – is examined in the light of the context of the wider traditions of practice which have shaped it.

Significantly, producing a critical appreciation of a piece of practice involves practitioners themselves in investigation of their own work, but as *part* of their normal duties and without the need to collect extensive data, or to take up extensive time using those resources usually needed for collecting or constructing, analysing, manipulating and presenting data 'objectively'. This is not to suggest however that in such appreciation there is no reference to wider thinking and writing. Neither does it assume that professionals will suddenly have additional time for this work, but rather that time could be found for professional self-study made public, from other activities currently aimed at feeding inspection and control systems. Further, such work redirects the focus of research by practitioners away from the arguably sterile concerns of both quality control and the Universities' Research Assessment exercises and instead recognizes practitioner research as serious self-study which can happen outside universities and inside professional practice (though of course fed at all levels, via libraries and increasingly through the Internet, by university research and teaching). That is, it is a proper *means* to professional development for those in practice and is properly carried out by practitioners themselves.

The rationale

If professional practice can, at least to some extent, be characterized as an art and the work of practitioners entails, *inter alia*, artistry (some of which is not just unquantifiable but also ineffable, mysterious, hard to express), then four things follow.

- Those processes useful for probing and understanding art from within the Arts should help practitioners to understand their professional artistry. (The processes of and language for critical appreciation can be made available to professionals who are prepared both to understand such approaches and to use them with due recognition of their provenance.)
- The artistry of our lived and felt experience as professionals and the understandings that arise from attending to these will be enhanced by being captured in artistic writing, because artistic expression is uniquely equipped to express the ineffable and the affective elements in our lives. (By attending to examples of art and artistry in life, art and professional practice, professionals can quickly become aware of what is involved in writing like this.)
- To be appropriate to its arts-oriented content, the writing that captures it should also be characterized by artistry in its presentation. (Practitioners thus need to be aware of and to utilize consciously the *artistic* elements of, for example, narrative, autobiography, form, structure, style and audience, and need to be willing to work through a number of drafts.)
- The resulting final portrait of a part of one's practice together with a critical commentary on the portrait and the practice itself, will then render the essence of the *particular* practice as a palpable and significant example of the practice of the profession,

seen within the wider professional context. (Practitioners can draw here upon the issues and principles of writing or reading a critical commentary in the Arts to enlighten the procedures for appreciating the artistry of professional practice.)

In summary, then, appreciating artistry in the caring professions may involve:

- recognizing elements which are significant in one's own particular practice;
- using the processes of critical appreciation to understand these elements better;
- drawing on knowledge about artistic presentation to enable the invisible, ineffable and tacit elements to be captured, made palpable and thus *become* part of the portrait of practice itself;
- standing back from this portrait and, by means of critical commentary, exploring the essence of the *particular* practice in relation to the practice of the profession.

The structure of the book

This book, like art itself, is intended to be responded to holistically. You are urged to recognize and respect the chronological nature of the structure here (both across and within sections) and not to skip around amongst them. (However, the fairly extensive references contained in some chapters are designed only for those wishing to pursue specific issues in depth.) The following offers the skeleton of the overall argument.

Part One

The first part of the book provides a basis for understanding the nature of professional practice in terms of artistry. Chapter 1 shows how – at a surface level and in public – there is much hostility, as the twentieth century closes, to the recognition and development of artistry in professional practice. This is not, of course, to deny the importance of the progress made in the technical and scientific knowledge which is used in or applied to professional practice, but to recognize that seeing practice in terms of artistry is equally necessary to professionals if their practical work with human beings is to be developed. A brief story about the dangers of proceduralization ends the chapter.

Chapter 2 looks at the artistry of the professional *in practice*. By considering specific examples of practice drawn from health care and education, it demonstrates – for those who are willing to see it – that professional practice even of this kind is better understood as artistry, and that it is the case whether or not practitioners themselves are aware of it.

Chapter 3 reviews the surprisingly extensive literature on professional artistry that exists across the caring professions, and looks at some of its characteristics as they emerge from this. A critical exploration of this literature shows that the writers are beginning to understand it better, that its importance has been recognized and that appropriate ways of investigating professional practice *as art* are now being sought.

If seeing professional practice as art is important, what kind of professional education might support, enlighten and develop it? Chapter 4 focuses on this central question and shows how by making critical appreciation a central process, professional development can be reshaped. This idea emerges from the fact that *artists* develop their practice and their ideas through critical appreciation of their own work and that of others, and by sharing and discussing such appreciations with colleagues. Such appreciation could also provide a valuable means of accountability – one which is more educational, more congenial to professionals and which would be cheaper than current bureaucratic processes. For example, professionals need to be able to explain their work specifically to fellow professionals, to traditional academics and to lay persons (including clients and the guardians of the public interest), and particularly need to use a language for this which is vivid and already universally understood. For these reasons response to and consequent recognition of the holistic quality of professional practice should arguably be at the centre of professional development.

The final chapter of Part One is focused on practitioner research. We have recognized that critical appreciation is a useful means of investigating professional work seen as artistry, and that, in this view, professional development and practitioner research become synonymous. Such research, then, needs to be supported by a paradigm which fosters rather than distorts it. But how can the appreciation of practice be supported and developed when all the current research paradigms are based on science and the social sciences? How, under such conditions, can critical appreciation be recognized as a serious research activity which enables professionals to establish a holistic view of their practice? One way forward is for practitioner enquiry to be reshaped and an arts research paradigm to be created – to function *alongside* (not instead of) the scientific, the interpretative and the critical research paradigms. The possible details of such a paradigm are suggested.

Part Two

Professionals wishing to discuss and investigate the artistry of their practice in detail need to develop a language appropriate to such a process and capable of being understood by lay persons. One such language has already been developed by those who write and think critically about the Arts. It therefore provides *one* starting point from which practitioners might develop their own language and processes for appreciating professional artistry. For this reason Part Two provides details of the language of appreciation of the Arts, by reference to specific examples of art. Chapter 6 looks at the narrative arts and the language for appreciating them, and thus gives us insight into ways of appreciating critically our practice and our writing about that practice. It considers in detail a story, a painting and a poem all of which relate to a well-known myth. But since the work of professionals is also substantially about performance, Chapter 7 explores the language endemic to the appreciation of the performance arts, and considers how and to what extent it can help us to talk about the nature of processes like improvisation.

Part Three

Part Three focuses on some practical issues which might act as a starting point for professionals seeking to investigate the art of their profession and the artistry of their practice. It provides a consideration of how professionals can begin to educate that discerning eye which enables them to appreciate and thus develop their own artistry, and that of their profession. Chapter 8 looks in detail at ways of recognizing and capturing the artistry of professional practice. Chapter 9 considers ways of presenting practice in draft form by drawing upon knowledge about and the language of arts appreciation as offered in Part Two. Chapter 10 looks at artistic ways of heightening the final portrait and at the reasons for doing this and Chapter 11 considers some principles which can guide the production of a critical commentary on the portrait and ultimately upon practice itself. However, writing an appreciation of professional practice is a creative act in itself, so only some broad principles can be offered here. How best to proceed in a given situation is then a matter for the writer's professional judgement and for his or her continuing discovery. Detailed examples are therefore not provided at this stage, but portraits of practice across a range of health care professions and a critical commentary on them can be found in Fish and Coles (1998).

The reader's role

The only excuse for seeking to take up a professional's time in reading about these matters is that the investment of effort in it will be substantially repaid. But how? Although our current world demands short-term 'answers' to improving practice, that is not what education is about. And so reading this book will not be repaid by an immediately improved efficiency in *practice*. Instead, it is an attempt to offer and explore a different *vision* of practice. And it can achieve little on its own. The only people who can change practice are the practitioners who carry it out. Education is about changing practitioners and particularly changing the way in which they *see* their practice. And that, above all, is what art offers too: new ways of seeing – new visions which compel and transform the beholder.

Part One

Appreciating artistry: new approaches to professional development and practitioner research

1
Contextual matters: art and professionalism

Introduction

Given the above definition of artistry, what is its significance? Why should practitioners be interested in it? What can it offer professionals, in a scientific era, who are caught up in the traditional demands of science and academe? This book seeks to consider the extent to which professionalism involves art and to show how practitioner research and development might be reshaped by focusing on artistry. As an introduction to these ideas, this first chapter examines the late twentieth century context for professional practice.

The chapter is offered in five sections. It considers first the extreme emphasis on science, technology and bureaucracy which has characterized the preoccupations and procedures of universities and professional accreditation bodies, the medical profession, politicians, economists, industrialists, the media and public opinion in Britain and many other countries in the last two decades of the twentieth century. Secondly, it notes the problems for professionals of their changing status in society as a result of the emphasis on science, technology and bureaucracy. Thirdly, it considers the evidence as the twenty-first century looms, of a new and gradual change in the way professional work is viewed, and sees this as resulting from discoveries that science, technology and proceduralization cannot be entirely relied upon. Fourthly, it examines in detail an example of the folly and inappropriateness of total reliance on bureaucratic procedures, science and technology in dealing with a unique practical problem where the overall situation was not 'read' and no one took a holistic view or drew upon an intuitive grasp of the circumstances. This story exemplifies the enduring need for professionals to draw on their artistry wherever unique practical problems have to be worked upon. It shows that professionals – like artists – need to be able to make new meaning out of what is happening within a practical situation rather than applying to it predetermined procedures. Finally, reasons are offered for claiming that the recognition of artistry and the improved ability to explain this dimension of professional practice are central to our defence of professionalism itself. And it is suggested that to collude in the denigration of the artistry of practice is to collude in reducing our own status as practitioners to that of sub-professional.

Empiricism in the 1980s and 1990s

The great achievements of science and the enormous capabilities of technology have, in the 1980s and 1990s, unleashed whole new ways of living and working. Technical tools and scientific modes of reasoning have characterized life in Britain and much of the world in these decades. So has the ideology of market forces. And of course these two major influences are inter-related. Indeed, it seems likely that in retrospect the late twentieth century will be seen as the technical rational age or the age of empiricism and materialism since almost every aspect of life is seen from within a strictly narrow version of reasoning and in empirical, materialistic and mechanistic terms. In this technical rational (TR) view, science is the only important subject, technology provides all the tools, bureaucracy sets up the required frameworks to ensure effectiveness, and market forces ensure efficiency. In addition, the false god of objectivity is worshipped and what is visible and can be quantified has real importance, while what cannot be expressed in league tables might as well not exist. In short, government and people alike seem to be mesmerised by data gathering, statistics and quantification, almost to the point of totalitarianism.

Evidence of this and of its influence upon practice in the caring professions is everywhere evident – so much so that it is already being accepted as the natural and inevitable way of living and operating. For example, government has intervened in all regulated professions to set up procedures to ensure efficiency. The language of the documents in which these procedures are enshrined is an indication of just how far this intervention has gone. Examples abound in every profession.

Part of this approach too is the superficially attractive but ultimately ridiculous demand that all practice should be evidence-based (best evidence being from controlled experimental work). Evidence-based practice (EBP) is currently a fashionable term in health care. It seems to have emerged from the notion of evidence-based *medicine*, which White (1997) has traced back to McMaster University in Canada. It is 'a systematic way of reviewing and evaluating the research literature in order to select the best intervention for a clinical problem. The research is evaluated according to its methodology and rigour' (see White, 1997, p. 175). This method of clinical problem-solving 'involves four main steps. Identifying the clinical problem, searching the literature, evaluating the research evidence and deciding on the intervention according to the evidence available' (White, 1997, p. 178). In one extreme version of this, one research team has worked to invent methods for distinguishing between testable and untestable assertions precisely because, they argue, decisions about spending need to be based on more rigorous evidence (Roberts, Lewis, Crosby *et al.*, 1996). They cite Health Visiting, calling for the reshaping of that entire profession because 'much of its nature and purpose . . . is expressed in untestable assertions . . . on which it is irrational to spend millions' (Roberts, Colin-Thomé, Crosby *et al.*, 1996, p. 27). Appallingly, there is in these arguments a real sense that anything which cannot be scientifically tested and measured could not possibly have value, and so at a stroke they call for the abolition of human and humane work.

It is as a result of all this that professional practice has come to be seen as a basic matter of delivering 'care' to clients through a pre-determined set of clear-cut routines and behaviours. The metaphor of 'delivery' is popular with those who take a TR view of professional practice, yet it hardly seems appropriate for describing the activities of working with patients/clients or pupils – activities which used to be characterized in terms of offering a service. We noted in Fish and Coles (1998) the distorting effect on how we see professional practice of the 'delivery' metaphor (pp. 31–32). We also noted that the ever present threat from accountability has been allowed to push the practitioner into such a defensive frame of mind that he or she is constantly in a 'no-win position', and how in essence it treats professional interactions as if they were industrial production systems.

The technical rational view of professional practice

Those who subscribe to the TR view argue that practice in the professions has for too long been surrounded by a mystique, and that goals can be set by society for professionals whose role should now be purely instrumental. They argue that the professional's role can be analysed technically and rationally in terms of activities and skills (though in the end this can tie things down further and further in the inevitably vain attempt to try to cater for all eventualities). They see improvement in practice (and quality) as incremental – as about moving on to harder skills (or competencies) and into more complex situations (but on a pegged resource base). Indeed, the fact that many of these competencies are simple and can be quickly taught, simply practised and easily measured or observed is also regarded as entirely desirable in a world of diminishing resources.

There has been then, at both a conscious and a subconscious level, a view that professional activities are essentially simple, describable, able to be broken down into their component parts (skills) and thus mastered. Here, a professional is one who puts into practice factual knowledge which has been learnt, in the theory classroom, from scientific research or as a result of new technology, and who follows procedures which his or her profession has established or which government has required. In this view, being a professional is about being essentially efficient in skills, and submissive in harnessing them to carry out other people's decisions. (This is to be contrasted with a view that sees professional work as involving practitioners who are broadly autonomous in the sense that they do not rely on others' ideas but make their own decisions about their actions and the moral bases of those actions.) The TR view of professionalism (which the work of Schön first highlighted) has prevailed in the late twentieth century.

The competency based view of practice, which is a logical extension of the TR view of professionalism, holds that practitioners are accountable for acquiring and operating a set of pre-determined competencies within a defined area of practice. This, however, suggests they are answerable *only* for skills and that all that matters is the technical accuracy of their work within the bounds of achieving other people's goals. This ignores (because they are less visible and less able to be 'proved' by means of empirical evidence) many other aspects of the professional's repertoire. And monitoring the practitioner's success is therefore about visible performance, simple observation and quick quantification. Some details of what this means in professional preparation and of how it differs from competence (a singular and holistic view of professional practice) can be found in Fish and Twinn (1997).

The language of quality control also springs from the TR model. It places emphasis upon visible performance and the practical aspects of the professional's work. It seeks to test and measure these, believing that technical expertise is all-important and that learning cashes out immediately into visible products. Thus the model is behaviourist, emphasizes fixed standards and quality control, and regards quality as measurable. It wishes to hold the professional practitioner accountable only for his or her technical expertise, and runs the risk of demotivating professionals by reducing their work to factory-like monotony.

Thus the TR view is a deficit view of professionalism since it is based on the belief that professionals will act ineptly unless they follow rules (often concocted by non-professionals!). It thus denies the real character of both professionalism and practice which in fact involve a more complex and less certain 'real world' where daily, the professional is involved in making many complex decisions, relying on a mixture of professional judgement, intuition and what – for the want of more precise language – we usually label 'common sense'.

Professional practice in a hostile world: the professionals' view

It is for these and the following reasons that in Fish and Coles (1998) we describe the situation that faces health care professionals in the later twentieth century as 'being under siege'. We also noted that prior to the 1980s it was somehow understood that 'what a professional actually does cannot always be pre-planned. The "right thing to do" emerges in the course of the professional's contact with patients or clients', that 'professional actions that require the highest level of expertise are those that simply cannot be predicted in advance'. We argued that professionals are educated and well paid because they have to 'make appropriate judgements in situations where there is no right answer', and where a moral dimension is involved (Fish and Coles, 1998, p. 4).

Such ideas were abandoned however because some professionals abused this trust. We pointed out that in the past malpractice was covered up by professionals, but that today any mistake can lead to legal consequences and professionals have become fearful of litigation. We added that by now too: 'a more educated and technologically sophisticated public no longer believes that professional work is so different from theirs' and 'is more prepared to ask questions of professionals and to demand answers' so that 'the mystique surrounding the professional has all but disappeared' (Fish and Coles, 1998, p. 6). We saw professional power reduced, and a general downgrading of professional tasks and status.

To increase the accountability of professionals was an obvious move by government. This led, in health care, to contracts which went way beyond the tacit understanding between professionals and their public, and in education has led to increased school inspections which have often got in the way of real teaching. This has left a legacy of competitiveness so that 'co-operation and collaboration', once key concepts of professional work, now seem outmoded and uncomfortable. Professionals' sense of vocation has been eroded (see Fish and Coles, 1998, p. 9). Health care guidelines and protocols have been developed, and in education the National Curriculum itself has been produced, in far more detail than in many countries, by bureaucrats attempting to ensure that professional practice is performed to the highest standards.

We also speculated that perhaps professionals have been an easy target because their work is often carried out intuitively and their knowledge of how to do it is tacit, and they 'would be hard pressed to explain their knowledge base for practising in a particular way or how they acquired the expertise to do so' (Fish and Coles, 1998, p. 8). We made the point that professionals are often isolated (in consulting rooms or even classrooms), they are single 'experts', expected to know everything, get it all right, make professional decisions of a high order and accept that 'the buck stops with them' (Fish and Coles, 1998, p. 9).

It is hard to know about cause and effect in some of this, but more recently some of these assumptions have been challenged. In close proximity to the millennium clear evidence is emerging – not only within the professions generally but in the public domain too – of recognition that professional work is not an exact science and that it can never be based solely upon science and technology but that it also needs a human dimension, which cannot be prescribed (and may even be driven out) by protocols, contracts and other government mandates.

Changing perceptions

Examples of such changes in perception can be found in the media (and thus amongst the public) as well as in the professional literature.

One powerful example in the public domain was the November 1996 television series *The Fragile Heart* – a television drama which explored rather more seriously than most, in a setting which drew on both Western and Oriental traditions of thought, some of the complex issues about the mind/body relationship and which opened up 'the mystery at the heart of the medical profession' by means of a heart surgeon's 'admission for the first time in his professional life, of uncertainty' (Dickson, 1996, p. A7). And while there are still stories from the media on what are seen as the 'flaws in medical practice', some writers have begun to argue the case *for* professionals against 'the view sedulously propagated . . . that the professions are a conspiracy against the laity' (Le Fanu, 1996, p. 4).

Further, many now within the professions are pointing to various examples of how technical rational ways of operating do not always bring the success once believed in. As far back as the early 1980s Schön was arguing for professional artistry and Capra was pointing out the need for a paradigm shift 'from the mechanistic to the holistic view of reality' (Capra, 1983, p. xix). Over a decade later Berwick complained that 'health care is in the midst of a love affair with measurement. Report cards, league tables, and mandatory reporting abound, all in a search for better accountability and an informed consumer. Belief in the wisdom of the market runs deep' (Berwick, 1996, p. 621). As a result, continuous quality improvement (CQI) and total quality management (TQM) have become hot issues. He points out that in the management view 'real change comes from changing systems, not from changing within systems'. The notion here is that bureaucrats should posit an ideal system, fix the funding and governance of it and then supply brief training to ensure that professionals operate as required within it. It was thought that this would show that professions can be improved by the intervention of government. But such interventions are already being seen as unsuccessful because they ignore the human dimension.

Evidence-based practice, as we have seen, is another example of a mechanistic approach. White (1997) argues strongly that nursing, being a young profession, would have difficulties with some aspects of it because there are vast areas of practice for which there is no research. She also points out that there can be philosophical conflict over what constitutes best evidence. She warns that the emphasis on EBP might limit the choices of nursing interventions available, that many nursing problems cannot be reduced to clear issues that can be resolved by scientific means, that EBP might be used to justify the restriction of choice of interventions, that the emphasis on EBP might disadvantage researchers applying for funding for non-experimental research, that it places at the bottom of the research hierarchy reflective research and reduces the authority of practitioners and the value of their experience. In examining the four stages of EBP she points out that many complex problems suffered by patients 'may not be amenable to reduction to a single clear question', that 'not all clinical problems are amenable to research' and that 'often ethical issues arise which require the delicate use of professional decision-making, codes of practice and the use of professional experience'. She also points out that this whole approach runs counter to another initiative in nursing – that of reflective practice. Making the point that aversion to EBP exists also in medicine, she cites Grahame-Smith's comment that EBP may be used as 'a means to shackle doctors and bend them to their managers' and politicians' will' (Grahame-Smith, 1995, p. 1126).

Examples of this kind of concern abound in health care literature. Ford and Walsh (1994) complained that the nursing profession 'has become obsessed with setting standards, yet this exercise appears at times to be little more than a modern version of demanding all the bed wheels be straight and all the pillow case openings facing the same way . . . . Unthinking regimentation is but a short step away from setting standards' (Ford and Walsh, 1994, pp. 96–97). Holmes (1991) noted the 'outrageous contraction of routine health services in order to fund prestigious, high-tech ventures of marginal value to the community'. He declares 'what we are left with are economic stringencies in the face of increasing societal need, i.e. a system which sees health care as a commodity, and the sick left to suffer because there is no bed, or because they cannot afford one' (Holmes, 1991, pp. 453–454). Hopkins and Solomon (1996), as researchers, argued against contracts in health care as 'unworkable control mechanisms and inappropriate vehicles for driving health care', particularly in areas concerned with chronic diseases and ageing. They saw the formal contract as a paper tiger (Hopkins and Solomon, 1996, p. 477–478). Beeston and Simons (1996) showed that experienced practising physiotherapists in a range of settings found theoretical models unhelpful in their practice, used more than neurophysiological and biomechanical frames of reference to help them understand their patients and their problems and were reluctant to identify with any one approach; that their 'starting point was the needs of individual patients'. Their practice was 'not premised on research findings or on any one theory' (Beeston and Simons, 1996, p. 241).

Holt (1996) and McMahon (1997) offer two examples of the extensive evidence of similar perceptions emerging from education. Holt, writing from an American university, but none the less an experienced headteacher in Britain, notes how 'current bureaucratic reform proposals overlook the need to address the way the curriculum experience is addressed in the individual school' and observes how 'politicians and administrators in most countries are obsessed with the notion of school improvement' (Holt, 1996, p. 241). McMahon, a teacher in a comprehensive school, writing in response to yet another attack on teachers by the Chief Inspector of Schools, complained that schooling in Britain today has come very close to Nazi Germany's purpose of education (which we found unacceptable earlier this century), which was 'to mould people to a fixed pattern, so that they are forced to fit in with the way of life imposed by a Government or Party'. He adds:

it is becoming clear that the real threat to education and its traditional values comes not from the soppily idealistic Sixties ... but
from the coldly cynical Eighties, when we were told that you
couldn't buck the market and that what was valuable could be
counted – and usually had a £ sign before it. What cannot be measured cannot have worth: what has no price has no value.
(McMahon, 1997, p. 32)

He added that 'Teachers have lost their commissions: they are all
NCOs now – National Curriculum Operatives, mechanical func-
tionaries of the state ... '. And continues:

A visit from OFSTED [Office for Standards in Education] demands
endless reams of paperwork from teachers who not only have to
teach, a task demanding enough in itself, but have constantly to
prove that they are doing so to the inspector's satisfaction by keeping insanely detailed records of their and their pupils' every movement. (McMahon, 1997, p. 32)

Clearly then there has been for some years a deep unease within
and across professions about the technicist and scientific approach
to shaping professions for the future, and also an awareness even
in the public domain of the lack of success of what Schön has called
'the proceduralisation of the professions' (Schön, 1983, 1987a).

Proceduralization: an example of its failure

Schön has argued that governments and public alike have
demanded that professional practice be reduced to a set of utterly
clear, simple, precise and easily implemented procedures governed
by controls 'designed to enforce [them] and to eliminate surprise'.
But they are now discovering the consequences of this – that however much tightening of procedures and controls takes place, surprises do not go away; that the strait-jacket that society has
imposed upon professionals to 'make them reliable' has not done
so.

I would wish to add that they are discovering further that the
indirect results have been strongly negative too. The worlds of professional practice have been demeaned, there has been loss of the
professionals' goodwill, a loss of creative thought, and a diminu-
tion in the willingness to take chances. This in turn has for example
reduced health care professionals' interest in that very on-the-spot

inventiveness which sometimes uncovers what it would take weeks of expensive tests to pinpoint. Further, for all the cost of the systems which have been set up, uncertainty has not been banished. It has, rather, simply been driven underground as something to which professionals hardly dare admit during their practice for fear of litigation. By contrast, the kind of professional development argued for later in this text uncovers and learns from uncertainty and requires few resources, provides real enlightenment and will still feed the current systems of accountability and quality.

The work of Schön offers a particularly graphic description of the failure that results from what he calls over-proceduralization and ignoring of the need for artistry. In a story drawn originally from Schön (1983) and offered to an English audience four years later (Schön, 1987b), he tells of the problems of near nuclear disaster at Three Mile Island in America. (This is also an interesting example of the power of one major art form – story-telling – to help us focus on important issues in professional work. Note, for example, how he makes the experience vivid by the repetition of the alarm signal, by the use of short sentences and by placing the reader in the action.) He takes his audience into the control room of the nuclear reactor, thus:

> There is a four foot concrete wall that separates you from the fuel rods, and you are looking at an enormously complicated array of lights, dials and gauges. The alarm rings. You must know that there are two sets of pipes, one that conducts water in direct contact with the fuel rods; the other, separated from the first, the secondary, that takes the heat from the first and uses it to make steam. The alarm rings, the pump kicks on in the secondary, the ... pressure relief valves open up, and the back-up pumps kick on to provide water to replace the water that has been lost.
>
> But it turns out that, unbeknownst to the operators, multiple errors occurred. The secondary pumps did not kick on. The light, designed to signal such a malfunction, was covered by a maintenance tag. Nobody saw it. The pressure relief valve did not close . . . . The light designed to indicate this, failed because of a lack of current . . . water began gushing out of the system, and some 30,000 gallons would be lost before ... the valve closed two hours later. (Schön, 1987b, p. 226)

Switching to reporting mode, Schön tells us that in watching their controls, the operators thought at first that everything was normal. Then they suddenly saw what they called 'a "Christmas tree" of alarm lights', and read on their dials what they later called 'weird data' of a kind they had never seen before. The situation was heading rapidly towards meltdown of a major nuclear reactor. At that point they were (as one of the operators later testified), 'riffling through the book of procedures to find the one that fitted the data'. They hit upon a (wrong) hypothesis of 'least damage' to which they clung for four vital hours. And as Schön says:

> Whenever there was a chance to interpret new data according to the 'least damage' hypothesis, they did so. There was a thud, for example, in the containment area. It could have been any one of three things: a change in the delivery of electrical power, a ventilator damper changing mode, or hydrogen exploding in the core. It *was* hydrogen exploding at the core, but the operators interpreted it as a ventilator damper changing mode. (Schön, 1987b, p. 226)

Schön says it reminds him of what they said at NASA (the National Aeronautics and Space Administration) when a rocket blew up: 'We did everything by the book and still it went wrong.' He later says this was one example of *proceduralization,* which he defines as 'attempts to reduce professional practice to a set of absolutely clear, precise, implementable procedures, coupled with controls designed to enforce them and eliminate surprise'. He adds:

> Underlying the systems of procedures and controls are theories; for such procedures depend on theories, for example, about the workings of nuclear reactors .... In addition, proceduralization depends on a theory of control: how to get people to do what you think they ought to do. These theories have to do with measures of performance and the use of carrots and sticks to make sure that practice conforms to the measures. (Schön, 1987b, p. 227)

Schön points up the irony of the consequences of proceduralization and control. The very designing of more and more procedures in order to ensure a perfect result is precisely what in the end gets in the way of efficient practice. He lists the following (which I have summarized).

- Whatever you do to eliminate them, surprises do not go away and there continue to be situations of uncertainty and unique cases – that is what professional practice is about.
- Because all that now matters is surface efficiency, people get to

be very good at not noticing surprise, at 'systematically avoiding attention to the data which if noticed would produce uncertainty'.

- They also invent 'junk categories' into which they consign that which they do not understand, in order to continue to believe in the adequacy of their procedures.
- Systems of control are multiplied when things go wrong, so that the procedures are increased and 'improved' – but never questioned.
- With increased systems 'we drive out wisdom, artistry and the feel for phenomena, all of which depend on judgement' and 'discretionary freedom'.
- We produce a world of 'increased routines and control and dubious achievement with respect to the disasters which we wish to avoid'.
- Games of control and avoidance of control emerge (managers devote a great deal of energy to the control of employees and employees to the avoidance of control).
- Keeping to the letter rather than the spirit of measures becomes the norm.
- The very system which has produced this becomes 'undiscussable' because people are being devious and this leads to the feeling of living in a house of cards which might tumble down if discussion did take place (see Schön, 1987b, pp. 227–228).

The need for artistry

This story and the comments upon it show the extent of the folly and inappropriateness of total reliance on the application of pre-learnt bureaucratic procedures, science and technology, in dealing with unique human, practical problems (and all problems have their human dimensions – even apparently technological ones). Scientific discoveries and technical know-how are of course useful, but the human dimensions of a situation – its inevitable uncertainties – are discounted only at our peril. We need to recognize, as does Eraut, that there will always be unpredictability and also that 'behind almost every precise calculation or logical deduction lies a set of assumptions that conceals doubt and uncertainty' (Eraut, 1994, p. 17). Knowing facts and how to apply them is undeniably useful for a professional practitioner. But all working practitioners know the importance of the ability to create new knowledge in situ and to be able to come to new understandings in new practical circumstances. Situations need to be 'read' – to be considered critically overall, not just accepted unquestioningly. Further, practitioners need to think critically and creatively, not to follow formalized instructions blindly. Their own assumptions in coming to the situation need to be challenged and a holistic or an intuitive grasp of the circumstances needs to be sought – and reassessed at various stages. During our daily problem-solving activities we need to keep in mind the whole and not be seduced into focusing in upon some small part of the situation in order to (or because we know we can) analyse and atomize it. The emphasis on what is known should not be allowed to mask from us the extent of our uncertainties, and the need to use them – in combination with intuition, sensitivity, imagination and creativity – to work on the problem. Further, in many situations it is not *uncertainty* that prevails but *indeterminacy*. Here the facts of the case are unavailable in principle because there is no logical possibility of the practitioner *ever* ascertaining them (Hunt, 1997).

On-the-spot responses to situations are then what professional work is about. It is also how artists operate. Further, operating procedures and protocols as if we were a mere agent of others is not only dangerous, but is also an acceptance of a sub-professional status and is demotivating. It is a subversive redefinition of our job by bureaucrats – perhaps to abrogate power to themselves and certainly to remove all those elements of discretion and of moral and practical decision-making which attracts people to join professions in the first place.

Conclusion

To recognize all these things is to accept the need for an improved ability to investigate, understand and explain all those matters that we have until now been content to refer to as common sense, or as tacit. Being articulate about the artistry in our practice is central to our defence of professionalism itself.

The real irony of all this (and the germ of a new vision) lies in the fact that the admission of uncertainty is actually the beginning of learning and development. Indeed, if professionals are to be freed to develop their practice fully, then the burdens of *being an instant expert*, of being assumed to know everything and of being expected to act speedily and always correctly and according to a pre-ordained 'book', need to be thrust off. They need to be replaced by *expertise* in and confidence about creating context-specific knowledge and developing professional judgements on the spot (see Eraut, 1994). These are educational, not administrative matters, and are developed by enquiring into practice and experimenting *as a part of practice* (see Fish and Coles, 1998).

Thus the defence and survival of professionalism itself is at stake where proceduralization is allowed to suffocate or deny the existence of artistry, and where artistry is not allowed to balance what science has to offer. Indeed, there is an urgent need for professionals to look in detail at the artistry of their practice in order to ensure that these vital balances are kept and to defend their professionalism. To explore and develop that artistry is to ensure that practitioners' work is – and continues to be – specifically defined as professional in nature.

2

Professional artistry: what sense does it make of practice?

Introduction

This chapter looks at professional artistry in the light of practice and at practice in the light of professional artistry, in order to understand both better. It is offered in two main sections. The first begins an exploration of professional artistry (PA) by presenting and discussing a piece of professional practice which has been designed and written specially to represent a common case of health care which involves practitioners from many professions, and which is also easily comprehensible by those in other caring professions. The second section focuses on two descriptions of practice, from articles which the reader will meet again in Chapter 3: that on nursing by Diers and that on teaching by Eisner. These are used to open up some ideas about how art can be harnessed to capture and respond to professional practice and thus how art can help us to understand practice better.

Exploring an incident from practice*

How you see it, how you don't

An illustration of perhaps the most obviously *technical* health care situation is of someone who suffers a broken leg. The task of the

---

* I am very grateful to my colleague Professor Colin Coles for constructing this exemplar especially for this purpose and for contributing to its subsequent discussion.

health care professionals is to set the leg appropriately, probably using a surgical procedure, and to allow natural healing processes to take their course. It sounds like a simple technical scientific matter. And if this is all that we *expect* to see in it, then it is likely that that is all that we shall see. (As is demonstrated by Schön's story of Three Mile Island, the TR view is sustained only by means of ignoring everything that challenges it. And the cost of ignoring or recategorizing everything which does not conform to this vision can be very high.) What underpins the PA view of practice then, is being willing to see practice anew. Being able to see anew depends upon being willing to do so, seeking to look from a deliberately different viewpoint and having the knowledge and language through which to make sense of what is seen. This involves 'reframing'. In Russell and Munby's words:

> Reframing involves 'seeing' or 'hearing differently', so the process of perception is a unified process in which observation *is* interpretative, and this is reflected in the language, in particular in changes in metaphors. (Russell and Munby, 1991, p. 165)

The frame through which the story of practice is seen and recounted, then, drastically affects our understanding of it. A sign of that reframing is to be found in a study of the figurative language used to capture it.

Further, the role the narrator has in the story also drastically alters that perception. It is easy to imagine the official reports on the following and how they might well imply that it was a simple input, throughput and output matter. On the other hand, it is also easy to imagine being any one of the various professionals involved and to recognize the complex human issues that arise for each one. Indeed, this whole story would be completely recast were it to come from the mouth and the mind of any participant from the ambulance personnel to the surgeon, from the nurse to the dietician, or from the patient to his relatives. Further, of course, the mind-set of the reader will affect what is heard, seen and attended to from the account. In all this, then, we are already dealing with three major elements in art – the cultural context from within which it is offered, the artist (narrator in this case) and audience (reader in this case) – all of which dimensions are also important considerations in capturing and understanding professional practice.

The following story, then, should be read with these questions in mind, from both the TR and the PA standpoint.

- What might be said about the *character* of this piece of practice?
- What might be said about the *way* this incident is told?
- To what extent are the processes involved in this incident shaped by TR procedures, and how important is this way of looking at practice to a professional who is trying to understand it?
- At what point and to what extent does the TR view of this practice cease to be useful?
- To what extent and in what sense is this exemplar of professional practice an example of PA and exactly how does the idea that artistry is involved help us to understand this practice better?
- At what point does the PA view of practice cease to be useful for understanding practice?

John: the case of the broken leg

John is in his early twenties. He rides a motorcycle. He is an electrician with a small firm of builders. He works in the North of the Country because that is where the work is. His home though is in the South, and his girlfriend whom he visits at weekends (when he's not playing football!) lives a two hour ride from his parents. One wet Friday evening travelling home he had a serious road traffic accident, and broke his right leg badly in several places.

The emergency services were soon in attendance. The police controlled the traffic. The ambulance people supported the broken limb, checked there were no further injuries, and decided John was stable enough to transfer to the nearest accident and emergency hospital. He was still a 100 miles from home.

John was in considerable pain. He was also concerned that he was already late. His girlfriend was expecting him. She would be worried. And his motorbike was a write off. If only he had taken out fully comprehensive insurance, but he couldn't afford it at the time. And he needed his bike to get to work. What was he going to do?

At the hospital John was thoroughly checked over in the Accident and Emergency (A&E) department, and his broken leg

X-rayed. He had only minor injuries otherwise. He was seen by the orthopaedic surgeon who was to set the fracture, and by the anaesthetist. The operation would be straightforward. The patient was young and fit. The surgery proceeded uneventfully, though the fracture was complicated and required internal fixing.

Postoperatively the nursing staff monitored John's condition, made adjustments to his medication and controlled his pain. John's girlfriend had been contacted. She would be coming to the hospital as soon as possible. His parents had also been notified. They were very concerned.

On the Monday morning John was visited by the physiotherapist. His mobility was maintained by exercising his healthy limbs. They discussed the physiotherapy that would ultimately be needed for the broken leg. The next day, John was also seen by the occupational therapist who discussed his home circumstances, his work, his lifestyle, and increasingly now an important concern for John, whether or not he would ever play football again.

Decisions soon had to be made about transferring John to his home town. He was torn about this. He would rather be near his girlfriend, but was well aware of his parents' anxieties. And his boss was asking when he might return to work. They had a big contract just come in that needed skilled people like John.

In due course, an ambulance transfer was arranged to take John to a hospital near his parents' home. There he continued physiotherapy and occupational therapy. He also saw the dietician as his physical inactivity meant he was rapidly gaining in weight. In due course the internal support to the broken limb was surgically removed. John's general practitioner visited him in hospital, and arranged for the practice nurse to visit him at home where he returned six weeks after the accident. Four months later he was back at work, but it was another year before he played football – he couldn't believe how long it took to get fit. He never did ride a motorcycle again.

The presentation of John's case

This narrative might be characterized as the story of a highly technical rational piece of health care practice, told in the clear, simple and factual language of a scientific account but without any recourse to technical terms. The discussion in the following section will explore the detail of the extent to which the practice presented in this story can be seen in technical rational or professional artistry terms. This sub-section will look at the way the story is presented. It is important during this discussion to remember that this story was written especially as a typical example of health care, by my colleague. He had no idea at all that the following details were to be part of the appreciation of his work – and the story is exactly as he originally produced it.

First, it is noticeable that John's story is told from an impersonal point of view by a narrator who uses the third person singular to refer to John and who is marginally privy to his thoughts and feelings, but who knows about the roles and witnesses the work of the health care participants in the story (and who enables us to do the same). And we are also reminded from time to time of the circle of people with whom John is concerned (girlfriend, employer, parents). This is, in literary terms, a story told by an omniscient narrator. The advantages of an all-seeing story-teller of this kind are of course that we, the readers, can see and be told about everything that the teller can know. Often this allows an exploration of a range of thoughts and feelings across many of the people in the story rather than restricting us to the viewpoint of the hero only. It can also lend an apparently 'objective', 'impartial' and even 'scientific' air because there is no one focal character who enlists our sympathies, and because as a result we are kept at a distance from everyone. In this story we are shown enough of John's situation – his worries and feelings – to enable us to imagine the human side of his story, while the health care staff are never individualized for the reader. We learn only of their profession and role. Indeed, we see them as a series of processes John has to go through. And we move in time with John through them, feeling his relative lack of control as he is passed relentlessly on to the next professional. Some days are named, some are not, reflecting the rhythm of John's awareness. We have a sense of the normal time scheme for this kind of case, but we also have a sense that for John this is how life is while he awaits discharge.

Interestingly the story begins in the present tense and turns to the past at the point where the accident happens. Although I think it is unconscious on the part of the writer, this beautifully captures the sense that just when life is going along normally (present tense), almost before you have realized it, fate has struck (past tense) and then ordinary living is irretrievably changed, disrupted, stopped, and life takes on a different, slower pace (also represented by a mixture of kinds of past tense). And all this, of course, reinforces our sense of the typicality of John's case – which after all is what the writer seeks to offer.

But if you look further, there are a number of simple structural and linguistic features which further support and contribute to this content. For example the sentences are all short. So are the paragraphs. And the language is almost entirely devoid of adjectives or any other 'subjective' language. There is in fact just one metaphor (and that a common, if slightly ironic one in this context), when the narrator says of John about the decision to transfer him back South near his parents' home, 'He was torn about this'. This both serves to highlight these feelings and to nudge us into a (perhaps subconscious) recognition that this story, though it shows compassion, and recognizes the human aspects of John's case, is otherwise very unemotional generally.

And finally, the cadences of the sentences also support the quasi-scientific character of this story which is both story and yet also nearly a report. (Cadence is the musical sound made by sentences and is produced by means of the way the words are emphasized and ordered in the sentence. Thundering rhetoric is produced by means of a considerable number of sentences, each of which is long, and made up of phrases whose length and sound is echoed several times within each sentence. Thus a pattern of sound is developed which is recognizable and which manipulates the listener into expecting and anticipating the rhythm, and waiting for the short end punch line. Further, the pitch and volume of the words fall towards the end of each sentence, like the pealing of great bells. A famous example is the passage from the King James Bible from 1 Corinthians 13, which ends 'but the greatest of these is charity'.) In the case of this story the cadences of the sentences echo the content. As the scene of the accident is described we sense the efficiency and routine surface of the drama in the short sentences with their level pitch, which might almost echo the quiet voices of the attending professionals. We hear through the middle section sentences which are even shorter, with a pitch which rises slightly at their ends because there is almost a question even in those which are not direct questions. This reflects the nervy worries of John as with mind whirling he thinks in staccato-like terms of all the things that would be happening to friends and family as a result of his accident. And towards the end, as things begin to sort themselves out, we hear longer and slightly more relaxed patterns of sound, where the natural sound the sentences make is of a long, slower, falling pitch, until there is a long and complex penultimate sentence (mirroring the regained complexity of living after the enforced simplicity of hospital life). This is followed by a final short shock. 'He never did ride a motorcycle again.'

Here, then, we have discussed something of the content, the intentions and the means by which the story is told. Clearly it deliberately stands back from offering the detail of professional work involved because it is merely a vehicle for helping us to explore the practice involved in this kind of case. To what extent, then, is the sort of practice represented here a technical rational piece of health care?

John's case and the artistry of health care

If it were to be characterized as a 'technical' piece of health care, the emphasis would be on clinical protocols and guidelines – sets of procedures – for the various actions taken by the health professionals. And indeed, for those wishing to see it only in this light, there is on the surface plenty of evidence to support this view. The emergency services, for example, will have followed a set of guidelines, so too would have those admitting the patient to A&E, and similarly with the operative procedures undertaken, the pre- and postoperative care, the transfer to the patient's home town, the rehabilitation, the primary care services. The staff involved will have received formal as well as on-the-job training to carry out these procedures. And further, the hard evidence for all this would be easy to find, and to record in impressive sounding scientific and formal language. Here, then, in a nutshell, is a neat, self-contained and apparently complete view of the case.

Yet for those willing to look beneath the visible TR surface at the particular and human experiences involved in this individual case, and who are willing to see it differently, there is much more. At each point during John's care (even from the moment when the ambulance was called), with every action taken by every health professional, procedures will have been subtly (or even greatly) modified to suit the particular circumstances the health professionals found themselves having to deal with – the uncertainties, risks and chances that were part of *this* situation. For example, no protocol will have been able to cover the individual nature of John's particular case. In making the myriad decisions about how and when to move and treat John and how and when to engage him in contributing to his own rehabilitation, all the professionals involved will have 'gone beyond the book' and called upon some creativity and imagination. In some way they will have improvised and even taken some risks, made new moves and responded to the particular situation. Some will have attempted to look at John holistically. Some will have empathized with John, some will have helped him to look ahead. Most will have thought on their feet, at some point, felt their way through the situation and picked up the subtler nuances about John's situation and his relationships. All will have striven to 'get it right', while doing a number of things at once. They will have learnt from and in the situation, theorizing as they proceeded. But the 'hard', direct evidence for this is less visible, more subtle and much more difficult to record directly, in scientific language.

The TR view is that by following protocols and guidelines, the necessity for health professionals to make individual judgements and take non-routine actions will have been minimized. It is also often believed that those judgements and actions that were necessary will have been made automatically and appropriately as a result of being trained to follow the book. However, the reality is likely to have been very different. The judgements and their resulting actions that the health professionals took in John's case will have been made, in the heat of the action, on the basis of very little information or may even have been made intuitively (drawing on what Benner and Tanner call 'an understanding without a rationale'; Benner and Tanner, 1987, p. 23). Beckett discusses these 'hot action' situations and describes the resulting judgements as marking out the work of a professional and as being critical in every sense (Beckett, 1996, p. 135). Further, very little of what happens to John during this story, and very little of what we see the professionals engaged in on his behalf is actually directed by evidence from scientific research. There will have been no time to search for such evidence and in many cases the research does not exist or is not conclusive. Indeed, the demand for 'evidence' may even obscure the importance of other kinds of knowledge. Worse, as Benner and Tanner point out, 'the most insightful and significant judgements may be overlooked, devalued or disbelieved because of an apparent lack of concrete evidence (Benner and Tanner, 1987, p. 29).

The practical knowledge used by all professionals in this event will have been that which has been learnt in previous practice or which is learnt during the event itself, rather than in classrooms or from books. There will have been various points at which professionals, in going *beyond* the book, will have been taking chances (because no one can know everything), thinking on their feet and doing many things at once. For example, the physiotherapists, like those in research reported by Beeston and Simons, are likely to recognize that the harmonious relationship that they establish with John 'may result in the therapist and the patient giving and assuming control at different times within the rehabilitation process' that 'models which lead to an analysis of practice on a purely biological or pathological level can be useful as a teaching tool for students, but do not adequately portray the realm of practice', that 'you have to learn to draw on everything that you possibly can because not everything works for everybody'. Like Beeston and Simons' respondents, the physiotherapist who treated John would have 'worked from a knowledge base that was a mix of formal and informal theories' (Beeston and Simons, 1996, p. 238). She or he would have been theorizing from practice in the situation, conducting subtle on-the-spot experimentations, trying out ideas with John about his rehabilitation, and how he perceived it and might contribute to it.

There will, too, have been tacit recognition by professionals involved that chance plays a part in all their work, from the proximity to the scene of the accident of the ambulance called, through the speed to which the patient could be operated upon, to the complications which could have accompanied the surgery. Elements of chance will have been reduced wherever possible, but – those who look at these matters will see – they can never be eliminated. For many of the professionals involved 'getting it right' will have been more important than going by the book. Perceptual skills, communication skills and creativity will have been harnessed to address this particular case. And everyone involved in John's health care will have improvised in situ at some stage in order to solve this practical problem and cope with its individual characteristics. But recognizing this improvisation will depend on a willingness to look beyond what is often dismissed as common sense or 'mere thinking on one's feet'.

Good professional judgement will also have been called for in John's case. Speed will have been of the essence at some points, deciding to do and doing will have been one action, perhaps, for ambulance crew, the surgeon and nurses. For example, the emergency service personnel needed to judge when and how to move the patient. In the A&E department, medical and nursing staff judged if other injuries were present and if so what tests might be needed to confirm this. (No patient ever receives every possible test on every occasion. Clinical tests and investigations are only undertaken when these are indicated by the particular 'signs' picked up by the health professional. These 'signs' are a complex mix of measurable and unmeasurable data about the patient's condition and circumstances.) Even during the surgery – perhaps the most apparently technical of all the procedures involved in this case study – the orthopaedic surgeon will have made judgements to adjust and modify the actions taken. Similarly, during the operation the anaesthetist, and postoperatively the nursing staff, will have made judgements and adjusted their actions based on their monitoring of the information they were getting not only from instrumentation but also from their observation of whether the patient was 'going off'. Perhaps even more so in the area of the patient's rehabilitation – in the work of the physiotherapist and occupational therapist, the dietician and of the general practitioner and practice staff – judgements will have been made to maintain the patient's motivation and to encourage self-help.

All these judgements would have involved a blending of the individuality of the circumstances (and the patient's changing circumstances at that) with routine actions which the health professionals had carried out in similar (though by no means identical) circumstances in the past. And because these matters are more subtle, the language which expresses them has to mirror this. That is why it is suggested that the language useful for appreciating art is what is needed here. But, of course, this whole view makes special demands on the political and administrative aspects of the caring professions and also on the education for professional preparation.

Professional artistry in the light of John's case

The case study then tells us a number of things.

- It shows the particularity of the individual situation.
- It portrays the way protocols and guidelines might be used as a basis for actions, but that what actually happens during the process of caring for a patient requires an interpretation by the health professional of these protocols and guidelines in the light of the circumstances at the time.
- It demonstrates that judgements (decisions about what to do) are made by all the professionals involved (whatever the status of the profession or the seniority of the staff). These are not all 'professional' judgements even when made by professionals. Some of these will have been intuitive (unreflective) judgements, some will have been strategic (a simple choice of skills and actions), some reflective (a more complex choice where skills, knowledge and capacities are called upon) and some deliberative (the result of moral consideration, and practical wisdom) (see Fish and Coles, 1998, pp. 280–281).
- It indicates that judgements are made even by non-professionals, such as the patient and relatives.
- It reminds us sharply that for care to be appropriate, there is a crucial need for a high degree of communication between staff, cooperation and collaboration, and coordination of the various elements of the care provided. This is the case not just in terms of the obvious and recordable actions undertaken (such as those written in the patient's notes) but also in respect of the less obvious and intuitive actions which probably are not recorded (or even which are unrecordable). In short, communication, cooperation, collaboration and coordination are more likely to be at a high professional level if the judgements of the staff are made explicit.

The case has also shown the range and complexity of the professional judgements made and actions taken in a health care situation, even though many of the actions undertaken will be covered by written protocols and established guidelines to which staff might have been expected to comply. If this quite legitimate 'departing from agreed practice' occurs in a case which is apparently highly technical (such as managing a broken leg), how much more is it crucial to understand the basis of the professional judgements made in other health care situations where:

- the diagnosis, management and prognosis are more uncertain;
- patients and relatives are key participants in the treatment process and must themselves make judgements (as in chronic disease such as diabetes or asthma);
- there is no active treatment at all, such as in palliative care.

We can see from all this, then, that the TR approach is not a measure of the degree of technicality of the processes involved. It is not something that applies more appropriately to some clinical conditions (like broken legs) rather than others (like chronic disease). Rather, it is a set of assumptions and beliefs *brought to how the case is seen*. The TR view involves *bringing* to the case the belief that health care can best be delivered through a narrow technical rational way of thinking, that there are sets of rules that can be identified (if we look hard enough for them) which, if followed unquestioningly, will deliver a consistently (and measurably) high standard of care (given sufficient training). But it must also involve an *unwillingness* to look at what challenges this view.

On the surface, then, John's broken leg might be characterized as a case requiring a TR approach to treatment – where practice might be seen as inevitably and *exclusively* TR. This is encouraged by the fact that the story of John's case is told from an impersonal viewpoint, by a distanced narrator who offers the barest of facts. Beneath this, however, at the level of the human condition of lived practice, the story can, arguably, also be seen in terms of professional artistry. PA takes a holistic view of practice, encompassing skills and the visible and quantifiable elements of performance, but also attending to all that lies beneath this visible surface. But it does not assume that all the judgements that professionals make are automatically appropriate, or that departing from clinical guidelines and protocols on a health professional's whim will inevitably lead to better health care. On the contrary, PA recognizes that all professionals at all levels make judgements all the time, and that health care practice rests on the appropriateness – on the moral and ethical as well as the practical nature – of the judgements that are made. It sees it as the professional's duty to be able to be able to articulate and explain his or her actions, giving due weight to their complexity. (By contrast, the TR view denies the significance, and even the existence, of such judgements.) In fact, such judgements are often made intuitively and on very little explicit information, and are difficult to recognize and to articulate without a language and a structure within which to do so. Much of the substance of this book is an attempt to offer one way forward on this.

The TR view of health care delivery, then, by contrast, makes the following assumptions:

- that health care delivery is only possible through the strict adherence to well thought out (and evidence-based) guidelines and protocols;
- that health professionals (especially junior ones, as lower status professionals) are not capable of making judgements (or should not be expected to);
- that professional judgements are dangerous departures from established procedures because they allow too much variability in situations that require to be controlled.

It also takes a more dogmatic and exclusive attitude to practice and to the development of it, being unsympathetic to any other ways of seeing practice and setting apart as irrelevant and inaccurate issues which challenge it. For example, this approach:

- ignores the existence of the judgements that all health professionals take all the time;
- denies the existence of artistry in practice;
- fails to recognize that high quality health care depends upon the good judgements of individual professionals;
- obscures the need for and the importance of professionals making explicit the basis of the judgements they make, and developing and refining them.

Unlike the TR approach, which seeks and values mastery, the PA view accepts the essential mystery of some aspects of human enterprise and behaviour. (Interestingly, Heath (1995) reminds us that 'mystery' was once a collective noun for doctors.) But this can mean that some elements of the artistry of practice are difficult to capture and discuss. Arguably, it is through the Arts and the processes of appreciating the Arts (which recognize what the artist has achieved) that the complexity and subtleties of professional practice can best be described. An artist is one who sees the world differently and uses abilities, means and materials to create 'a work of art [which] throws light on the mystery of humanity' (Emerson, 1982, p. 47). Or, as Bullock reminds us, 'an artist can give to a particular moment of vision caught in a poem, painting, play [or narrative], a universal significance . . . the experience looked at and felt from the inside' (Bullock, 1990, p. 665). In this sense professional practice involves artistry both in itself (the professional practitioner can be seen as an artist in meaning-making in the practical setting) and in various responses to professional practice (practitioner as story-teller about practice and enquirer into practice).

Artistry and appreciation

In this view, to improve practice is to consider it holistically, to work to understand its complexities, to look carefully at one's actions and theories as one works, subsequently to challenge them with ideas from other perspectives, and to seek to improve and refine practice and its underlying theory. In this way, as Stenhouse (1980) pointed out, an artist (musician, painter, poet, novelist, dramatist) also works to improve practice.

Artists do not simply follow rules, and similarly the PA view of practice sees it as starting where the rules fade (because the rules rarely fit real practice). Art relies on frameworks, and rules of thumb rather than protocols. It works with interpretation of details, acknowledges the inevitable subjectivity of setting them down, and seeks an understanding of human activities by means of recognition and response. This recognition and response is exactly what is involved in the process of critical appreciation in the Arts and in professional practice. Artistry seeks room for creativity and recognizes the need to take risks. Artistic activities (by comparison with craftsmanship) involve the practitioner not only in skilled routines but in wider abilities and capacities, particularly open capacities which by definition are never able to be mastered. It involves doing the unexpected and doing it well. It sees the practical situation as a whole and practitioners as being in dialogue with the situation (see Schön, 1987b, p. 31), just as an artist *discovers* his or her content and form *as he or she works*. The professional artistry view sees professional practice as an art in which risks are inevitable, where learning to do is only achieved by engaging in doing together with reflecting upon the doing, and where improvisation, enquiry into action and resulting insight by those involved in it *generate* a major knowledge base.

By looking anew at the practice involved in the example of John's broken leg, by seeking to confront those dimensions of it which we usually try to ignore, and by probing beneath the surface of procedures and common sense, it does seem possible to gain some understanding of the expertise of professional practice which is otherwise obscure. And one useful way of capturing and considering those aspects which involve the professional in operating like an artist is to draw upon what we know about art and artistry, and particularly critical appreciation. Indeed, perhaps there is enough here to lead us to believe that professional development itself is actually about the further development of artistry.

Professional artistry in practice: some implications

Professional artistry, then, is not merely about writers finding aptly figurative language in which to express their insights about professional practice. Rather, practice itself *is* a form of art and practitioners are a particular variety of artist. This means that practice can be understood in artistic terms and that professionals operate in the same way as – use the same processes as – artists in fields like music, painting, poetry and dance. It is therefore appropriate to discuss professional artistry in the language used to discuss the Arts. However, this does not mean merely making pragmatic reference to one of the Arts drawn upon in an off-the-cuff way in order to solve an occasional problem in understanding and articulating some aspect of professional practice. Instead it means understanding the way artists themselves work and also being familiar with the ways in which the Arts are appropriately discussed and explored, and using this in a properly disciplined way to improve our understanding of the artistry of practice. This in turn means seeing professional practice holistically, as an art, though it does not mean seeing it *only* from this point of view.

How, then, can art be harnessed to capture and respond to professional practice and its artistry? In the following section we shall note some aspects of the nature of art and consider two extracts which utilize language from the Arts to describe some aspects of the nature of practical knowledge.

Capturing professional artistry: how can the Arts help?

Art, artifice and truth

One of the paradoxes of art is that artists use *artifice* in order to capture vividly and to get closer to understanding better some aspect of life *as it is lived* (some truth about the human condition). For example, fables like Æsop's about the tortoise and the hare, and parables like the New Testament story of the Prodigal Son, are invented and embellished constructions from an imagined world which, though fictional, carry great truths.

Thus poets, for example, who have a vivid and fresh vision of something significant about an aspect of life – or love – which they wish to capture, explore and share, often turn to complex and artificial structures to help them to express and clarify it, or, more likely, they discover as they struggle to capture and refine what it is that they want to say, that a particular poetic form emerges from under their pens and then somehow demands to be worked upon and worked within. The conventions and traditions of that form then operate as a discipline within which (or against or even beyond which) the poet strives to clarify what he or she is trying to say.

For example, the sonnet has evolved as one of the most highly contrived poetic forms, traditionally consisting of fourteen lines and with some conventional ways of structuring this overall unity. Within this the poet can set up one of several expected rhyme schemes and these, together with rhythm, punctuation and layout, are used to shape this 'little sound', which originally came from Italy, into groups of lines – perhaps seven couplets, or an octave (eight lines) and a sestet (six lines) or three groups of four lines and a couplet. To be successful, as a poet works over various drafts, a poem *evolves* into a sonnet where each of these elements of composition works in a harmony which is particularly (even peculiarly) appropriate to the content (the shape of the statements, questions or arguments) of the poem. There were too, in Renaissance Italy and England, certain expectations by the reader of the sonnet in respect of subject matter, language, attitudes expressed, poet's voice and reader's response. The Petrarchan and Shakespearean sonnets evolved at this time, and courtly love, by convention, saw the unattainable, distant and often disdainful lady addressed in poetry by a desolate lover doomed to failure by status and position at court. The traditional subjects of the sonneteer were love and death. But neither form nor subject were imposed on the poet in a technical rational way and later poets used this tradition differently, relying on the reader to recognize that the earlier conventions had been flouted. Thus George Herbert (startlingly) wrote religious sonnets to a distant God in the very terms and form used earlier to woo courtly ladies, while John Donne wrote both secular and religious love sonnets; and some of Hopkins' sonnets were truncated, consisting of only 10 lines arranged in proportion according to the original sonnet structure.

There is something special about the overall unity of a sonnet. It expresses its ideas appropriately in the tight discipline of very specific schemes of rhythm and rhyme, and uses, within its miniature framework, 'poetic' language in which more is implied than is said and from which the reader can take further the ideas – the figurative language – begun by the writer (where the metaphors and similes bear the weight of extension). Its striking vocabulary, vivid images and deliberately reshaped syntax, are all recognizable as part of the charm of the piece, but do not constitute the entire nature of the poem. In other words, while a sonnet is made up of these elements, there is more to it and it has more to offer the reader than can be understood simply by analysing or summarizing them. Readers willing to give it some attention will find this revealed in any Shakespearean sonnet (which can be found at the back of most editions of the Complete Plays) and are particularly directed to those with famous opening lines, such as 'Shall I compare thee to a summer's day?' (sonnet XVIII) or 'Let me not to the marriage of true minds / Admit impediments' (sonnet CXVI).

What is significant about all this, however, is that the demanding and highly artificial form and conventions of the sonnet are used by many poets to capture and express universal and simultaneously highly individual and personal – and often very deep – thoughts and feelings. They offer us new visions of an aspect of life – our own life – which once seen, we all believe we always knew, and which the reader responds to with a quivering recognition. And, again paradoxically, sometimes it is the very artifice of the sonnet that has enabled the poet (the maker, as the Greeks called such a person) – and us the reader – to distance ourselves from *and at the same time come closer to* the experience or vision offered. This enables the poem and its experience to affect us deeply and it recalls and makes reverberate for the reader previous similar experiences and half-seen visions. Thus, when a poem achieves that shiver down our back, it is often because at a conscious *and* a sub-conscious level the poem was written and we now read it *as a unity*, and as almost magically recreating for us that vision or experience. Of course it would be possible to look at the rhythm and rhyme, the form and structure, the language and mood, the metaphor and simile that make it up, but when we have done so we shall no longer be responding to art but categorizing it scientifically and we shall not have captured all it has to say and all it could offer us. The reverberations of vocabulary, imagery and meaning come from somewhere we shall still not have put our finger on, and will echo and be pursued onwards in our minds well beyond the end of our reading.

Thus, too, the apparent artifice endemic to writing about professional practice, where the writer has deliberately sought out and explored colourful ways of expressing – sometimes indirectly – a new vision of what it is like, may well also be an aid to understanding that practice better. This is a far cry from the demands of empiricism of course, which seeks truth and 'hard' evidence, validity and reliability of a piece of practice, and which seeks (via analysis) to atomize it – to break it down. By contrast, writing which draws upon art and artistry to explore professional practice offers elements that the writer and the community share only at a sub-conscious level, and some that the writer or reader is only dimly aware of, and which is only validated by a quiver or shiver of recognition from the reader. The artistry of professional practice then deserves to be recognized, responded to and captured in ways like this. During this capturing the writer needs to exercise artistry in representing justly his or her original vision. A critique of that capturing of practice can then respond to both the artistry of the original practice and the artistry of the writer.

Thus we have a threefold process in appreciating professional practice, which is as follows.

1   The sharp recognition of some aspect of practice (which others may have overlooked) which (as a result of focusing on and enquiring into that practice) is seen anew by the writer, and which has both individual importance for the writer and also some more universal significance for readers.

2   The capturing of this vision in a carefully chosen and much worked over portrait, where the writer discovers more about the practice and his or her vision of it *during* the attempt to capture and do justice to expressing what has been seen. During this capturing process, new language may have to be drawn upon, language different from that usually used to talk in empirical terms about professional work, just as a poem uses language removed from ordinary discourse. This writing thus often becomes more contrived and apparently increases its distance from the lived practice, and yet paradoxically thus comes to express it more fully and accurately.

3   The creation of an appreciative response to what the writer has captured, which recognizes the vision and something of the way the writer has worked to capture it, makes somewhat more explicit what has been achieved in the writing (which underlines and explores further what the writing has encapsulated), and responds to its value to individual practitioners and perhaps even to the profession as a whole.

With these ideas to help us, then, let us now consider two descriptions of professional practice, one from health care and one from teaching – both from America – in order to explore the artistry of the writing and to consider what it can tell us about professional practice and whether or not this sort of writing offers something useful and new, enlightening and persuasive. They will certainly be found to be in great contrast to the 'reported' case of John's broken leg.

Professional artistry captured: two examples

Diers (1990) writes in artistic terms not about a specific piece of nursing practice but of nursing practice generally. How then does the language and how do the references to art which she employs contribute to her and our understanding of professional practice in nursing? She draws attention to the self-discipline which underlies nursing (and the Arts), and neatly attaches the idea of discipline to the idea of professional practice by adding that it is discipline that makes a person practise, as dancers or opera singers do. Here she both asserts and demonstrates one element of similarity between art and professional practice and gives a further emphasis to the word 'practice'. In order properly to keep the distinction between art and professional practice clear, however, she says: 'the tool of the nurse ... is not the body or voice but the intellect, exercised on human problems and possibilities'. (One of the essences of successfully employing language to indicate similarities between two things, lies in not losing sight of the differences between them.) Thus, successful metaphors (where one thing is referred to as if it has become another) or similes (where one thing is described as 'like' another) depend upon keeping both aspects in view (see Diers, 1990, pp. 65–66).

Diers says that nursing practice is not 'a matter of learning the script of a play, then rehearsing and repeating it'. Rather, she argues, using a striking metaphor, 'nursing is choreography'. And she explains that in part this means seeing the nurse as 'balancing demands gracefully, attending to the tunes others play, and moving in synchrony with the *corps de ballet* ' (Diers, 1990, p. 65). So does this language draw attention to something significant about nursing, and if so how successful is it in conveying this? Does this metaphor bear the weight that is placed on it and can it be extended further beyond what she says here? Certainly the picture painted by these words is impressionistic rather than literal, it offers no hard evidence for what it says but asks us to draw upon our senses of sight and sound to validate this description from our own experience while at the same time we recognize that we had not quite seen nursing in that way before. For example, it captures vividly at a surface level the attitudes to others that are part of nursing and implies more than it says in capturing the calm, almost gliding and yet speedy movements of the professional nurse, the all-important awareness of others and the essentially responsive nature of some aspects of the nurse's work. These are all key (and well known) elements of nursing. But this writing makes us see them in a different vision, where the central image of a ballet dancer is created by implication and yet is supported by every part of the description used, and which adds up to a sort of caricature of nurses' everyday practice, but which is at the same time entirely sympathetic to it. It is hard to imagine how these subtleties could be recognized, captured and conveyed by any other means. Such a description is, then, very useful in thinking about these character-istics of nursing – even at the level of raising important issues about what is the nature of nursing practice.

And this is not a one-sided and unbalanced vision of a passive professional. Diers adds, putting her finger on two major elements of any art – the pattern and the form:

> But on another level, the nurse as choreographer moves others. She decides what pattern and form are important for patients and then moves people, machines, paperwork and decisions . . . . A clinical nurse specialist moves a physician consultant slightly to the left, walks with a head nurse to stage right, and moves the clinical investigations committee downstage, dictates the dance they will all do to the music chosen, and then stays out of sight behind the cur-tain. (Diers, 1990, p. 65)

To show that the overall imagery of this passage can bear further weight, and that the amusing yet serious caricature can be taken further, here we have a different metaphor from the same overall analogy, and a new scene on the dance stage. Here the comparison is not between nurse and dancer but nurse and designer of the dance. And this metaphor is usefully extended to help explore the nurse's proactive role. Diers' imagery neatly makes the patient the central focus, the object 'being danced to' (and the phrase 'dancing attendance upon' comes to mind). And she provides us with a modern dance sequence which is directed by the nurse and which is made up not only of real people but of also paperwork, machines and decisions – all of which we see dancing before us in a complex, almost cartoon, pattern which simulates the busy-ness of life in the ward. This deliberately 'mannered' dumb show then gives way to a scene – almost a dream sequence – in which the nurse directs overtly (but from behind the bed-curtain) a number of the physical moves which in real life she no doubt often longs to do but which she can only do very subtly, if at all. That is, she takes hold of the consultant and shifts him or her to the side, moves very deliberately with the head nurse to place him or her in a dominating position, and by directing them downstage, distinctly lowers the status of the bureaucratic procedures.

This seems vividly to capture the actions, motivations and feelings that can be part of the daily practice of nurses. The fact that it is done lightly and with humour, underlines rather than detracts from its seriousness, and perhaps enables some things to be said that it would be difficult to say in other terms. And these images linger for far longer with the reader than might many a statistic.

Taking the analogy yet further, Diers also points out that:

> the nurse-choreographer's talent is to create, out of the moving bodies, the electricity of conflict, the stirring music of commitment, a piece of action that is whole and intact, smooth and integrated, subtle as a minuet or rowdy as a polka. (Diers, 1990, p. 66)

And here she has almost bitten off more than the language can chew. There are perhaps rather too many differing images coming at the reader. The first half of the sentence seems to lead in one direction and explore the theatrical and musical means of creating (or sharpening the import of) a piece of drama, while the second picks up important issues about the unity of art as being more significant than its constituents and the third tries to round up (and see holistically) the whole dance analogy by characterizing two interestingly different dances. This is not an economic piece of writing for all that it takes up fewer words than it takes to summarize it, because it does not hold together. It is impossible to know whether this is an example of some good ideas run rather too much into each other to make the impact that they deserve, if it is the product of a fierce editorial hand, the cramming of several sentences together to fit a required number of words, or a belief that the reader might not be able to take any more! In any case, the rest shows (by contrast to this last sentence) that this sort of writing, to be successful has to be worked over, and that when it is, it can be very powerful.

By contrast to Diers' work, Eisner's early attempts at working on artistry in teaching by *likening* teachers to artists saw him using simile instead of metaphor, music instead of dance. (It is interesting to note that by comparison with the vivid immediacy of meta- phors – for example, 'teacher is artist' – which sweep the reader into quick acceptance that teacher is at one and the same time a teacher and an artist, similes imply a more hesitant approach and invite a more thoughtful response – 'teacher is, er, um, *like*, um . . . an artist'.) Sometimes, however, the writer is more beguiling and starts with a tentative simile, slipping quietly to the assertion of metaphor once the reader has been caught up in the language! In seeking to reinstate the importance of the art and craft of teach- ing in America in the early 1980s, Eisner published an article which is lavishly illustrated with striking black and white pictures that emphasize his central image that teachers are, in their work with classes, like orchestra conductors. Here he was seeking to offer robust opposition to an apparently popular view that education is a science, which was part of the political climate of American schooling at that time (and which his descriptions make sound remarkably like our own present circumstances).

In this provoking article he claimed, with supporting examples, that 'teachers are *more like* orchestra conductors than technicians. They need rules of thumb and educational imagination, not scient- ific prescriptions' (my italics) (Eisner, 1983, p. 4). He goes on to argue that the art of the teacher appears most clearly when working on a question and answer session with a class.

He pinpoints the moment in that teaching session where the teacher does not quite know what to do next (an experience that will be familiar to every teacher – of children and of adults – and irrespective of the detail in which they have prepared their teaching). Eisner then shows how the teacher reads 'the muted and enigmatic' faces, the body language, the contextual signals, of the class and indicates how sensibilities come into play which allow the construing of the situation. He refers to this as the educational imagination coming into play in considering options (that is, although he does not say so, operating professional judgement). He talks of the teacher thinking 'on her feet in many cases *like* a stand-up comedienne' (my italics) (Eisner, 1983, p. 10). He then adds (slipping deftly from similie to vivid metaphorical language) that what we do in this sort of situation:

> is to orchestrate the dialogue moving from one side of the room to the other. We need to give the piccolos a chance – indeed to encourage them to sing more confidently – but we also need to provide space for the brass. And as for the violins, they always seem to have a major part to play. How is it going? What does the melody sound like? Is the music full enough? Do we need to stretch the orchestra further? When shall we pause and recapitulate the introductory theme? . . . How can we bring it to a closure when we can't predict when a stunning question or an astute observation will bring forth a new melodic line and off we go again? (Eisner, 1983, p. 10)

Here, again, the analogy between teacher and conductor is stretched to provide us with a scenario we recognize all too well if we have taught. The shy members of the class (characterized by the high-pitched and nervous piccolos), who need a space made for them, the solid reliable ones who always help a question and answer session along almost as if you had paid them beforehand to feed you the next line (characterized by the endlessly busy stalwarts of an orchestra, the violins), the noisy ones (the brass) who often speak before they have thought but who need to be helped to recognize this weakness in order to learn, are all neatly encapsulated in the various instruments described. So far, the description perhaps does little more than put in fresh language what we already know. But the orchestral image does force us to see the unity of all this, rather than the individual elements, and further, it does help us to feel free to admit and to explore the crux of the professional judgements that have to be made at this moment. The short questions are important here. They still use the central musical analogy, but now they do more than make us feel comfortable because we recognize the scene. Now the imagery captures the difficulty of knowing the right moment to move things on, to press further, to go back, to repeat, to bring this part of the lesson to a conclusion. They concentrate our attention on the risks we have to take and the endless possibilities that we shall cut off something important not only for one pupil but for everyone including the teacher, that a new version of the melody might lead to fresh improvisation and catch the understanding of someone who has missed it all the first time round. In all the work on professional judgement in teaching, it would be hard to find a passage which better exemplifies this moment of judgement.

Deliberately coming out of the vision he has created in order to reinforce the seriousness of his point, Eisner adds:

> Clearly teachers are not orchestra conductors. Yet teachers orchestrate. The analogue rings true. Is artistry involved? Clearly it is. But where does it occur and of what does it consist? (Eisner, 1983, p. 11)

He concludes (with ideas which Schön later echoes) that it occurs when the rules fail, when new forms of teaching that were not previously part of our existing repertoire have to be created on the spot. The need for this is, he says, recognized by means of attention to pattern and expressive nuance. In response the teacher must be able to 'call on or invent a new set of moves' that 'create an educationally productive tempo within the class'. This involves risk-taking. Such response, he argues, represents the apotheosis of educational performance which is rare and to which we ought to offer a seat of honour. He contrasts this with the craftsperson as a performer within the rules. He argues for the space for teachers to be free to respond creatively and talks of the aesthetic in teaching as being 'the experience secured from being able to put your own signature on your own work – to look at it and say it was good'. This comes for example, he says, from students discovering the power of new ideas, the satisfaction of a new skill learnt or the intriguing dilemma of an intellectual paradox understood. It means being swept up in the task of making something beautiful. He argues that these aesthetic moments in teaching are among the deepest and most satisfying aspects of educational life. He recognizes that this is an 'unabashedly romantic image of teaching' (Eisner, 1983, p. 12) and an ideal to which we should strive. None the less, he leaves the reader understanding much more about how, in practice, artistry can be used to explore professional judgement.

It would seem then, that recourse to the language and ideas of art has a role to play in helping us to understand some of the subtleties of professional work. But it is important to ask whether these examples are mere aberrations or are part of a tradition of thinking. How substantial, then, is the notion of professional artistry? How extensive is the current literature on professional artistry? Is there 'critical mass' behind this notion?

3

Professional practice as art: mirage or vision?

Artistry as a major characteristic of professional practice: current evidence

Although the prevailing climate has been and to some extent is still hostile to artistry, there are professionals in all areas of the caring professions who have over many years both recognized professional artistry and argued for it. This third chapter demonstrates the extent of the field and explores critically some of the resulting literature. It considers writings from the multidisciplinary field of education for the professions, and from five major professional areas within this (the medical profession, nursing, physiotherapy, occupational therapy and teaching) and it makes brief reference to Traditional Chinese Medicine. By attempting to address the following three questions it considers in what ways professional artistry is more than a mere shibboleth (or is a vision rather than a mirage). It asks these questions.

- What is actually said across professions in this literature about how professional artistry is defined and characterized?
- What is the significance of the ideas in this literature about professional artistry, what light do they shed on professional practice and how relevant do they seem to be in understanding and improving professional work?
- What seem to be key issues and common themes across this literature?

The following exploration inevitably attends only to a sample of what has been written. It has been chosen because it represents views across a fairly broad spectrum of practitioners, professional educators and researchers. Firstly, some literature is considered whose main subject is the nature of professionalism itself and/or professional education generally. Because it tends to be read across all professions, some of it has been particularly influential in offering a common language and some widely shared ideas about professions as arts. Secondly, health care literature is explored for views about the artistry of practice. Thirdly, teaching and teacher education are considered. The literature in both these latter two sections tends to be read within rather than across professions. All sections are presented chronologically in order to reveal the development of ideas, and brief consideration is given in each section to the issues and themes which occur across the literature of that section. Readers are urged to read all sections irrespective of their particular professional interests since each profession has something to offer to and something to gain from this survey.

As will be seen below, in some cases the term 'professional artistry' is used fairly loosely in these writings. At this stage therefore it would be premature to try to define it in exclusive terms. A further examination of the concept is therefore reserved for Chapter 4.

Literature from the field of education for the professions

A number of important writers have discussed the nature of professionalism generally rather than as part of the practice of a specific profession. In doing so they have done much to shape the thinking about professional artistry. Some (like Freidson, 1994) have seen the definition of professionalism as an issue in its own right. Others (like Schön, 1987b, and Eraut, 1994) have been concerned to explore the nature of professional knowledge as a basis for professional education. Some (see, for example, Higgs and Jones, 1995, and Fish and Coles, 1998) have begun to work with colleagues in cross-professional ways to examine professional knowledge. By drawing upon work that has influenced professions generally, this review provides evidence of the very way in which professionals in a wide range of fields regard and discuss their work.

Defining professionalism

In the literature on teaching, Hoyle (1974), in writing which still
has relevance today, offered ways of characterizing the restricted
and extended professional, and Langford (1978) offered a view of
professionals as existing only as part of a community. But it is the
work of Freidson on professionalism which has sought to reconsider its spirit and to reconcile it with the world of the very late
twentieth and early twenty-first centuries. He makes the point that
the idea of professionalism is generally about performing 'complex
discretionary work' (Freidson, 1994, p. 10), but that there is no
simple definition which will 'win the day' for professionals in the
present hostile world (Freidson, 1994, p. 27).

It is perhaps in the notion of the *discretionary* nature of work
that ideas about professional artistry have taken root. In emphasiz-
ing choice, decision-making, autonomy and thus creativity, Freidson suggests that professions in all cases are:

- occupations within higher education;
- where there is a commitment to the occupation itself, to fellow
  workers and to clients (see Freidson, 1994, p. 126).

Considering the knowledge and skill, motives and meanings, values
and commitments endemic to professions, he says that the work
professionals do, being 'esoteric, complex and discretionary in
character', 'requires theoretical knowledge, skill and judgement
that ordinary people do not possess, may not wholly comprehend,
and cannot readily evaluate'. For this reason, he adds, 'the clients
of professionals must place more trust in them than they do in
others' and professionals must honour that trust and accept that
clients' needs must take precedence over the professional's need
to make a living. He indicates that a professional's work is 'very
important for the well-being of individuals or of society at large,
having a value so special that money cannot serve as its whole
measure' (Freidson, 1994 , p. 200).

Freidson then summarizes professional work as:

- involving a 'commitment to practising a body of knowledge and
  skill of special value and to maintaining a fiduciary relationship
  with clients';

- requiring a 'relatively demanding period of training in order to learn to do esoteric and complex work well';
- developing (as a result of education) a commitment to knowledge and skill so that a professional's work becomes a central life interest which provides its own intrinsic rewards;
- being concerned as a result of this with extending and refining their work within the broad commitment to maintaining its value to society;
- actually identifying themselves with the skills they exercise so that what they do is not solely for the income (see Freidson, 1994, pp. 200–201).

These attempts to clarify the nature of professional work focus far more upon the human interaction involved in professional work and its resultant responsibilities and demands than upon the specialist knowledge and skills required (though of course it does not ignore these). Freidson makes it clear, as do all those who write about professionalism, that first and foremost professionals work with clients and in doing so must act in response to whatever situation they find themselves in. And no situations of this kind are ever totally predictable nor can there ever be pre-formulated rules, processes or theoretical knowledge which will be simply and neatly applicable in that situation. From this point of view, it may be that professional work does require something akin to artistry since central to it is the need, in response to the particularities of the situation, to create, 'on the spot', a response which is in some respects entirely new. It would thus seem that the motivation to see professional work as involving artistry comes from the very nature of professional work itself. But this still does not define professional artistry, nor tell us much about its role and place in professional work. The work of Schön helps us to begin to understand this better.

The notion of professional artistry

The name of Donald Schön has in the late twentieth century been connected specifically with the notion of reflective practice and with demonstrating the arguments for eschewing a technical rational approach to professionalism (in which he uses the Three

Mile Island incident related in Chapter 1). But it is in bringing the idea of professional artistry to our attention that he has perhaps rendered professionals the greater service. In the introductory chapters of his seminal work *The Education of the Reflective Practitioner*, he offers examples drawn from a very wide range of professional contexts, of how professional practice can be acquired. He begins this work by explaining professional artistry thus:

> I have used the term *professional artistry* to refer to the kinds of competence practitioners sometimes display in unique, uncertain, and conflicted situations of practice. Note, however, that their artistry is a high-powered, esoteric variant of the more familiar sorts of competence all of us exhibit every day in countless acts of recognition, judgement, and skilful performance. What is striking about both kinds of competence is that they do not depend on our being able to describe what we know how to do or even to entertain in conscious thought the knowledge our actions reveal. (Schön, 1987b, p. 22)

This last sentence is crucial to understanding artistry in its recognition of a key problem which affects professional development as well as research into professional activities. The *knowledge* involved in our knowledgeable actions is tacit and difficult to bring to the surface, is difficult to formulate and do justice to in simple words. This also makes it difficult to convey to others, and hard to utilize in order to explain our actions or to explore professional activities, so we use words like 'common sense' instead. But since the Arts specialize in communicating ideas, thought and feelings which are usually regarded as tacit or even ineffable, we have here the beginnings of reasons for linking the artistry of practice with work in the Arts.

Schön characterizes the operation of artistry in professional settings as: engaging in a dialogue with a unique (particular) situation of professional practice. (Schön's term 'unique' is somewhat inaccurate here since, as Golby points out in relation to case study, if a situation were unique we would have no means of relating it to anything else and no way of understanding it or working on it (see Golby, 1993, pp. 7–8).) Schön suggests that professionals work within the traditions of their profession and follow the rules of enquiry into that kind of practical problem. But, as he points out, this also involves going well beyond those rules and (taking

account of the traditions of the profession), inventing on the spot
and testing new rules, new methods of reasoning, new categories
of understanding, strategies of action, ways of framing problems
and new experiments. These he says are central to professional
artistry (Schön, 1987a, pp. 36–39). Here the practitioner behaves
'more like a researcher' (Schön, 1987a, p. 35). He says:

> when practitioners respond to the indeterminate zones of practice
> by holding a reflective conversation with the materials of their situ-
> ations, they remake a part of their practice world . . . (Schön, 1987a,
> p. 36)

The artist, of course, is quintessentially a 'maker', who operates in
just this kind of way (although of course the converse is not true –
it is not the case that *any* maker is an artist).

It is clear here that for Schön professional artistry is expressed
in everyday parts of a practitioner's work. For him, the individual
and particular situations which require such artistry occur not
rarely, but all the time, and thus the very definition of a professional might be one who deals with situations for which there can
be no simple book of rules or rigid training. In referring to professional artistry then Schön is describing a kind of knowing which is
in (endemic to) the action being carried out. For him it is clear that
the professional needs to understand the traditions of practice in
his or her profession, to know those rules, processes, skills, abilities
and capacities that are the norm for working within that profession, and to be well aware of the traditional ways of operating in
practice and the appropriate methods of enquiring into it.

The artistry then, lies in knowing when and how *to go beyond*
those rules and traditions (not ignore or deny them but to continue
the evolution of the traditions of that practice) and in being able
to create something new in response to the individual situation,
having 'read' it without preconceptions and having interpreted it
from outside the tyranny of routine thinking and assumption.
Noting that this is a matter of understanding the nature of professional knowledge, Schön quotes the philosopher Ryle to indicate
that procedural knowledge involves doing *one* thing (knowing *as*
doing) not two things (knowing and *then* doing). This virtuosity
(the ability to do, to think and to act *as one ability*) in practice,
lies at the heart of two key problems for professionals: how to help

people learn and develop such practice, and how to explain it and defend it in the public arena. Eraut is one writer who has offered some help with these.

Practical know-how and the nature of professional knowledge

Schön offered us some important starting points, but some of his ideas are not very fully worked out. Gilroy (1993), Eraut (1994, 1995) and Beckett (1996) have offered sharp criticism of his work. Eraut says it is not practical enough, being useful only at a meta-cognition level and offering ideas about ideas rather than starting with actual practice. In writing about educational matters for professions generally, Eraut makes the point that the processes of learning practical knowledge are little studied and little discussed (Eraut, 1994, p. 14). He characterizes the kind of professional knowledge which Schön calls artistry as 'practical know-how, which is inherent in the situation itself and cannot be separated from it' (Eraut, 1994, p. 15). He, like Schön, notes that much of it is inevitably tacit.

Eraut turns to parallel examples from the Arts to help him to illustrate the difficulties in capturing and transmitting the knowledge that makes up professional practitioners' *activities*. This 'procedural knowledge' (or as Oakeshott says, 'practical knowledge') involves the truth about matters *for the person involved*. It is to be contrasted with the propositional knowledge (factual or scientific knowledge) where scientific truth is a concoction of a group, and thus is a matter of greater objectivity, being easily written down, conveyed to others and tested (see also Oakeshott, 1962, p. 146). Eraut notes that unlike scientific knowledge, the knowledge embedded in a piece of music, a painting or a dance cannot be fully represented in words. Knowing the 'meaning of the signs, symptoms and the "feel" of a particular patient in a particular situation is neither readily encoded nor transmitted as a process to another practitioner'. Eraut adds: 'There are important distinctions between awareness of tacit knowledge, subjecting it to critical scrutiny and being able to articulate it in propositional form' (Eraut, 1994, p. 15).

He also draws attention to what he calls 'the problem of uncertainty which pervades a great deal of professional work'. He adds that much professional work is characterized by 'wise judgement [made] under conditions of considerable uncertainty'. He also makes the very important point that 'a significant proportion of the learning associated with change in practice takes place in the context of use' (Eraut, 1994, p. 33). He therefore argues against professional education courses where knowledge is acquired first and 'used' afterwards and points out that 'Not only does an idea get re-interpreted during use ... but it may even need to be used before it can acquire any significant meaning for the user'. He also believes that learning professional practice is made the more difficult because 'there is little immediate transfer of learning from one context of use to another' (Eraut, 1994, p. 33). These ideas deeply challenge many courses for entry to individual professions.

Taking the thinking about these issues further, Eraut notes the following.

> Some kinds of practical knowledge are uncodifiable in principle. For example, knowledge which is essentially non verbal: the tone of voice or a musical instrument, the feel of a muscle or a piece of sculpture, the expression on a face cannot be fully described in writing. Verbal performance, such as teaching or advocacy, which are not fully scripted beyond a brief set of notes, cannot be reduced to simple technical descriptions. (Eraut, 1994, p. 42)

Here we see the first of many attempts to explain or understand the operation of professional work in terms of artistry. Rather than fighting against or trying to eradicate uncertainty, these approaches (unlike TR approaches) accept it and try to understand its nature. But are the notions of artistry, and the ideas drawn from the Arts merely useful analogies whose significance is limited to the odd occasions when they are employed, or is artistry actually endemic to professional practice? Does the work of a professional *involve* artistry? Is artistry a defining characteristic of professional practice or merely a useful source of illuminating metaphors and similes to be employed briefly to aid understanding?

Eraut certainly goes some way towards answering this. He frequently refers to the creative aspects of the work of a professional, the need for intuition and 'the need for invention and insight' (see Eraut, 1994, p. 113). These are the same characteristics commonly regarded as essential also to artists themselves, and so Eraut seems certainly to be suggesting that professionals *are*, to some extent, artists and not merely *like* artists. However, seeing professional practice in this way is a matter of values and beliefs, a matter, like beauty itself, of what lies in the eye of the beholder and, indeed, of what determines the very choice of where to look. Such seeing may also be related to one's preferred cognitive style (divergent thinkers, for example, being naturally more able to take on board ideas about artistry, convergent thinkers being naturally more happy with a technical rational approach). But even if this is so, it could not reasonably be argued that professionals should operate inflexibly in only one mode. Indeed, the ability to see their practice from a number of different perspectives is central to the professional's ability to generate creative solutions to unexpected problems.

What Eraut and Schön have shown us, then, is that it is entirely possible to see professional practice in terms of artistry, and thus to argue that something more than a mere figure of speech lies behind phrases like 'the art of medicine or nursing or teaching'. What, then, is useful about seeing professional practice in this way? How far have these ideas been taken up? To what extent are they able to be taken up in the present climate? Consideration of the literature in health care and education yields some answers to this, but so too does some recent cross-professional work in this field.

Artistry and professional judgement in health care: cross-professional work

Professional judgement and its near relative, clinical reasoning, offer an interesting case in point. Of three recent edited collections on cross-professional work which attempt to look at these issues (which are central to professional practice), the first (Dowie and Elstein, 1988) is concerned almost exclusively with a technical rational view of professional judgement. The second (Higgs and Jones, 1995) takes a practical rather than a technical rational standpoint on clinical reasoning, and at least nods in the direction of artistry, while the third (Fish and Coles, 1998) concerns itself exclusively with the professional artistry of professional judgement (whilst not denying the contribution to professional practice of technical rationalism). Citing three books (one of which this reviewer has co-authored) does not of course demonstrate a trend. But it does serve to indicate a development in direction.

Dowie and Elstein's edited volume (1988), then, contains chapters designed to bring the techniques of scientific research to bear on issues like systematizing human judgement, and even on what is called the art of diagnosis (which turns out to use theories of probability to investigate 'models of steps towards diagnosis') (see Eddy and Clanton, 1988, p. 201). Higgs and Jones (1995), while they recognize that 'professional practice involves science/technology, art and craft and the use of the corresponding forms of knowledge' (Higgs and Jones, 1995, p. xiv), none the less rarely mention art and artistry and these do not appear at all in its index. The editors do however claim towards the end that the book offers 'a view of clinical reasoning in which all types of knowledge are valued' and it does list amongst these 'studying and expressing knowledge through literary texts, visual art and drama' (Higgs and Jones, 1995, p. 314). But none of this is pursued in any detail.

The attitude to artistry to be found in the earliest of these three books might be summed up in the chapter by Dawes in Dowie and Elstein. She says:

> Friends tell me that important human judgement is often ineffable, unsystematic, and intuitive.
> I agree. And it is, therefore, often bad.
> Friends tell me that decisions that are effable, systematic and explicit decisions are dehumanized decisions.
> I agree. But they are 'dehumanized' only for the decision-maker, and I am concerned with the consequences for the people affected by the decisions. Bad decisions are dehumanizing for them. (Dawes, 1988, p. 150)

She argues later:

> in a wide variety of psychological contexts, systematic decisions based upon a few explicable and defensible principles are superior to intuitive decisions – because they work better, because they are not subject to conscious or unconscious biases on the part of the decision maker, because they can be explicated and debated, and because their basis can be understood by those most affected by them. (Dawes, 1988, p. 151)

Here intuition is *asserted* to lead to less good decision-making than decisions that rest upon a few principles, which, although Dawes does not say so, are *chosen subjectively and defined from a viewpoint which is itself subjective,* without acknowledgement of that fact. Here are the usual claims that the technical rational way, the way of thinking which embodies a logical, scientific and technical approach, is unassailably objective, while everything else is subjective and thus inferior. Some of these arguments win the day because practitioners (even those who acknowledge artistry in their practice) neither challenge them, nor refute their TR nature by laying bare their inherent subjectivities. Neither is there yet any widespread systematic attempt to explicate and deliberate about 'intuitive decisions', which is what I am arguing for.

By contrast, Fish and Coles (1998), which includes the work of colleagues across medicine, nursing, occupational therapy and physiotherapy, explored the operation of professional judgement via ways of appreciating practice. Here, we were attempting to understand better the essentially human and artistic nature of professional practice. Our work was centred on reflective case study examples of practice in health care and the specific actions and judgements involved in them. We saw these as characterized by professional artistry. The professionals, with whom we worked over a one-year period, were able to uncover and understand better their practice and themselves. Each individual professional's path through his or her enquiry was different. Yet there were principles and processes in common across these cases which demonstrably enabled practitioners to see, in their practice, issues ignored by the TR approach. It is the *processes* used there (of appreciating the nature of professional practice and understanding its living detail) which are considered in greater depth in this present book.

Recurring issues and themes in the literature on education for the professions

There seem to be two key issues in the literature reviewed so far: the nature of *practical* knowledge, and the creativity central to professional practice. The nature of practical knowledge is shown as complex, difficult to learn, needing to be better understood by practitioners themselves and their clients, but in some cases as *uncodifiable* in principle. However, this seems pessimistic. 'Codifying' suggests a TR process of constructing rules. Practical knowledge, however, *may* well be able to be *expressed* (codified), by artistic means. The creativity endemic to professional work is about 'going beyond the book'. Professional practice is unpredictable and uncertain (working with people in a morally responsible way whilst seeking their good involves treating each situation as particular). These issues show professionals working more like artists than scientists, but also show them ill-equipped to talk about this expertise although they operate it daily. Setting out to explore this daily practice using more artistic forms of expression may be a way forward. The case studies of professional judgement in health care are a striking example of this. In order to pursue this in detail it is now necessary to turn to the profession-specific literature.

Profession-specific literature

Artistry in medicine and nursing

In Western medical practice and in nursing, there is much literature from the past which shows how, in the early stages of their development, both these professions were regarded as characterized by artistry and actually referred to as an art rather than a science.

In nursing, for example, Nightingale wrote: 'Nursing is an art but if it is to be an art, it requires as exclusive a devotion and as hard a preparation as any painter's or sculptor's work; for what is having to do with dead canvas or cold marble compared with having to do with the living body, the temple of God's spirit' (Tooley, 1910, p. 123). Hampton notes that 'nursing originated as a household art and later developed into a vocation' (Hampton, 1994, p. 15). It is she too who reminds us that 'between 1900 and 1940, efforts were made to clarify the professional status of nursing', and she quotes Rew's suggestion that 'this focus on developing a profession of nursing with a distinct body of knowledge led to an emphasis on the science rather than the art of nursing' (Rew, 1990, p. 30). But, in fact, as Carper notes, in America at least, 'the term nursing science was rarely used until the late 1950s (Carper, 1978, p. 14). This dependence on science to provide the credentials for claiming professional status is found commonly in emerging professions throughout the twentieth century. But ironically, the technical rational aspects of scientific thinking seem, in most health care professions, to have become the rod with which to beat them and the very means by which the public and governments can reduce their status to that of sub-professional.

Medicine too came into the twentieth century seeking status from science and many doctors tried to hold on to the arts aspects in the face of the power of science. Schweitzer (a doctor of music before he was a doctor of medicine) wrote of a doctor's duty being to remember that medicine is an art as well as a science and high-lighted the art involved when the individual doctor interacts with the individual patient (see Mole, 1992, p. 113). And the spirit of this was carried on in America from the 1960s when the *Journal of American Medical Association* began to reproduce fine art on its cover and to present essays on art and medicine (see Southgate, 1997). But of course there are repercussions when doctors admit uncertainty, as Katz reminds us. The work of doctors, he admits, is engulfed and infiltrated by it, and there is still 'uncertainty whether to base the practice of medicine on modern science or ancient art, or both'. But he refers to clinical judgement as 'the practice of the art of medicine' (Katz, 1988, p. 558). Heath's monograph on the 'secrets, mystery and particular contribution of general practice' (Heath, 1995, p. 4), is even more emphatic. Having pointed to the destruction of vocation by market values, the conflict between advocacy and distributive justice, and the spe-cious separation of health care and social care, she argues that general practitioners 'need the ability to identify imaginatively with a wide range of individuals'. She adds that they must:

> make available the benefits of scientific medicine but mitigate its dangers through an understanding of anthropology, biography, poetry, myth, philosophy and politics. The skills of anthropology and biography help us with empathy and the use of continuity and an awareness of poetry and myth can help us find the words to communicate our understanding to the patient. (Heath, 1995, p. 35)

One way of finding the words of course – and of examining one's practice in more detail – is to put one's practice into stories and to capture it in critical incidents (see, for example, Benett and Dan-czak, 1994; Bradley, 1992; and Pringle *et al.*, 1995).

But it is in the literature of nursing that these ideas are more prevalent and are explored in more detail. The following section looks at *some* of that literature which exemplifies the struggle to understand professional practice as art. Because of lack of space, it draws in the main on literature from Britain and North America.

Nursing literature, 1978 to 1990

Carper's four fundamental patterns of knowing

The work of Carper (1978), although written from within an American context in the 1970s, is still recognized in the 1990s in Britain and America as an important basis for thinking about artistry in nursing (it was described in 1994 as 'now one of the most widely cited articles in nursing': Chinn, 1994, p. viii). The assumption in all citings I have seen is that Carper has set an important foundation for nursing in exploring these issues. But we must ask at the very end of this section just how beneficial that influence has been.

Carper (perhaps not surprisingly) seems to struggle to be specific about what she calls 'the open texture of the concept of art' in nursing, but she proposes four fundamental patterns of knowing (or ways of thinking about phenomena) in nursing. They are: the empirics, the science of nursing; the 'esthetics', the art of nursing; the component of personal knowledge; and ethics, the component of moral knowledge in nursing (Carper, 1978, p. 14). Interestingly Carper notes the reluctance in nursing to recognize an artistic way of knowing, and complains: 'one is almost led to believe that the only valid and reliable knowledge is that which is empirical, factual, objectively descriptive and generalizable' (Carper, 1978, p. 16).

Of the art of nursing she says: 'There is, nonetheless, what might be described as a tacit admission that nursing is, at least in part an art'. But she adds, 'not much effort is made to elaborate or to make explicit this esthetic pattern of knowing in nursing' (Carper, 1978, p. 16). Her attempt to be more specific about what the art of nursing means includes the following (summarized) ideas.

- Art is expressive rather than merely formal or descriptive.
- An aesthetic experience involves creation and/or appreciation of a singular, particular, subjective expression of imagined possibilities or equivalent realities which resist projection into discursive language.

- It leads us to acknowledge that genuine knowledge and understanding is considerably wider than our discourse.
- The art of nursing is made visible through the action taken to provide whatever the patient requires to restore or extend his ability to cope with the demands of his situation.
- The art of nursing is expressed by the individual nurse through her creativity and style in designing and providing nursing that is effective and satisfying.
- It is creative in that it requires development of the ability to 'envision valid modes of helping in relation to results that are appropriate'.
- It relates to the whole patient and total care.
- It involves empathy – the capacity for participating in or vicariously experiencing another's feelings.
- It is about knowing particulars rather than a class (see Carper, 1978, pp. 16–18).

She sees the design of nursing as needing to be accompanied by 'a sense of form, the sense of structure'. As Holmes (1991) notes, she thus 'posited aesthetic knowing as the highest form, in the sense that it was concerned with the balancing and integration of the other forms, and with acting in relation to projected outcomes' (Holmes, 1991, p. 451).

Carper concludes that nursing depends on 'the esthetic perception of significant human experiences'. But these are rather vague notions of what artistry in nursing involves, and thirteen years later the writing of Holmes was still calling for real clarification of these matters. What Carper has usefully done here, however, is to establish firmly the notion that art is 'a way of knowing' which is different from ways of knowing in, for example, science. What she has perhaps less helpfully achieved is the turning of attention to 'esthetics' rather than to examples of art itself (although she does refer to specific examples of issues in art, like balance and rhythm). She does not define 'esthetics', but she clearly sees it as concerned with ideas *about* art rather than ideas drawn from the study of specific art. In producing what has become a seminal article in nursing, then, Carper may have helped the thinking about ways of knowing, but she may also be responsible for some of the failure to ground later thinking about the artistry of nursing in *art* itself. Indeed, she may have been responsible for directing some nursing scholars' attention to the aesthetics area of the continuum which runs between aesthetics and specific examples of the Arts.

Artistry and intuitive knowing
In the 1980s in America and Canada, several writers in the field of nursing explored intuitive knowledge, by following up the work of Carper. Of these, Benner's name is the best known. Working with Wrubel in 1982 she highlighted the importance of feeling in the repertoire of nurses, noting that 'the perception that something is wrong [with a patient] often begins with a feeling' (Benner and Wrubel, 1982, p. 12). They also cited Polanyi's notion that some people possess skills (including the ability to make qualitative, critical and discriminating judgements) that are irreducible to objective measurement. Such characteristics, they claimed, are found in expert nurses. They argued for the development of nursing expertise of this kind, and Benner's classic publication extended this idea that intuition is the hallmark of expert nursing (Benner, 1984), although it takes an unsupportably hierarchical view of experience (implying that novices have no relevant experience), and uses TR language and ideas.

By 1987, writing with Tanner, Benner argued that 'intuition appears to be a legitimate and essential aspect of clinical judgement'. She adds, trying to explain in TR language and without recourse to artistic vocabulary, that 'intuition is defined here as *understanding without a rationale*. Such an understanding is not a mystical or accidental human capacity. Intuitive judgement is what distinguishes expert human judgement from the decisions or computations that might be made by a beginner or a machine' (Benner and Tanner, 1987, p. 23). This article also notes, again without exploring this in artistic language, that 'pattern recognition is a perceptual ability to recognize relationships without pre-specifying the components of the situation' (Benner and Tanner, 1987, p. 23). In their sense that perception is indeed holistic, they echo both the individual work of Agan (1987), and the overall therapeutic approach of Traditional Chinese Medicine. Although they do not say so, seeing holistically is also characteristic of artistry and of the Arts themselves (see Chapter 6).

Benner and Tanner add later that 'commonsense understanding is a deep grasp of the culture and language so that flexible understanding in diverse situations is possible' (Benner and Tanner,

1987, p. 35). And they note, significantly: 'the most insightful and significant judgements may be overlooked, devalued or disbelieved because of an apparent lack of concrete evidence' (Benner and Tanner, 1987, p. 29). They make the point that: 'it is not nursing's fault that we distrust intuitive judgement based on a deep background understanding. A mistrust of knowledge other than formal mathematics has been handed down in the Western tradition since Plato' (Benner and Tanner, 1987, p. 30). They also note that 'neither information-processing nor statistical-decision theories are particularly useful in describing how an expert clinician zeros in on the right region for assessment, selects what is relevant from the vast field of clinical data available or recognizes changing relevance as the situation unfolds' (Benner and Tanner, 1987, p. 31). They end with the following warning which echoes Benner's 1984 publication:

> Unfortunately, Western culture in general has proposed replacing intuitive judgements with rational calculations. Rational calculation, apparently, is being confused with human reasoning and is being mistakenly proffered as the epitome of knowledge. One consequence of this mistake is a false dualism: analytic reasoning versus mysticism. But intuitive knowledge and analytic reasoning are *not* an either/or opposition; they can – and often do – work together. (Benner and Tanner, 1987, p. 31)

Writing at the same time as Benner and Tanner, but in Canada, and acknowledging Carper's and Benner's work, Agan also argues that intuitive knowing is a dimension of nursing. He centred his investigations on holistic nursing, gathering material from a qualitative study of the perceptions of intuition of seven 'holistic nurses'. (These are nurses who base their work on holistic medicine.) He reports how they describe the use of a non-rational, intuitive way of knowing in their practice, and argues that this might contribute to 'a change in the state of nursing art' (Agan, 1987, p. 63). By recording their metaphors for intuition (some of which are in fact drawn from science), he shows how nurses think about it. He noted the following: 'making connections like an electric current'; 'therapeutic touch' which enables them to reach deeper into the person; 'opening themselves up' and 'using antennae'; 'feeling attuned'; and 'feeling it in my skin'. He concludes, surprisingly, that intuitive knowing is a form or dimension of personal (rather than aesthetic) knowledge, referencing this to Carper (Agan, 1987, p. 70). Apparently feeling the need to legitimize via theory what he has discovered from practice, he comes back to Carper's categories, which do not particularly extend his ideas here.

The excitement of discovering more about the artistry of nursing for the 1980s then was, at least for some, about recognizing intuition as a formal component of nursing. Issues about intuition were also pursued in the 1990s, but along rather different lines. By then, some more detailed references to the Arts themselves were offered and deeper questions were beginning to be faced, including the central issue of defining the meaning of artistry in nursing. The interesting articles of the 1990s still seem to emanate from America, but at the same time there begins to be a growth in British writing – which is a response to the work of Carper and of Benner and her colleagues (see for example the collection of nursing stories in the *Nursing Times* in September 1991 (volume 87, number 36) and January 1992 (volume 88, number 1)).

Nursing literature of the 1990s

Art and the artistry of nursing

Diers – a small part of whose work we examined in Chapter 2 – takes a bold and original approach to these issues. She notes that 'nursing is so enormous ... that no metaphor from any one art can encompass it' (Diers, 1990, p. 66). She offers an instructive and refreshing attempt to define the artistry of nursing, by trying to draw distinctions between the art and craft of the profession and by turning rather more directly to art itself. She argues that the search for beauty motivates the clinician as much as the painter or musician, offering as evidence the idea that 'cure is more attractive than disease, and belief more beautiful than confusion; logic is lovelier than irrationality, and order is more decorative than chaos'. She makes detailed reference to drama and music and argues that 'nursing changes with each patient, each situation, even each heartbeat' (Diers, 1990, p. 65).

It is noteworthy that amongst the rather more erudite literature, this work seems at first sight rather less scholarly. However, that says more about what we expect and are used to from articles about professional practice than about the quality of this work. In fact it not only gains much in shedding the impersonal formality of standard journal articles and writing more directly about nursing as art rather than dressing it up as aesthetics, but it probably represents rather more closely the thinking of many practitioners. And it is not less scholarly for focusing on these matters. Indeed, it offers new ideas, critical consideration of which might well take forward our thinking about professional practice. Diers' work, then, shows clearly that a new language is necessary for discussing the art of practice. What we have to do with writing of this kind is to probe the metaphors (as we did in Chapter 2) to see how far they really help us to understand aspects of professional practice, and whether they genuinely do direct our attention to something which has not been and cannot be expressed in any other way.

But if this article is an example of those that attempted to consider matters from a more practical standpoint, still much of the nursing writing of the early 1990s (now British as well as American) operated at a theoretical level, perhaps because the ability to deal with matters at the abstract level was assumed to be a necessary aspect of the very scholarship which nursing was trying at this stage to build up.

In what sense is nursing an art?

Holmes (1991) sets the more international scene well for this part of the story. Indeed, Gray and Pratt (1991), which contains Holmes' work, is much more positive about the artistry of nursing and the future possibilities for investigation and clarification of it. Holmes points out that using nursing theory as a stepping stone to establishing a science of nursing has been a political matter and has been about establishing professional autonomy. Alluding to what I would argue can become a very sterile debate, he notes that:

> most nurse theorists concede that nursing is both an art and a science, and some place great value on the artistic component, seeing it as the dimension which adds quality to technical proficiency. But where is the understanding of nursing as an art expressed in nursing theory? We are beset by problems when we insist that nursing is an art, and yet nurse theorists have consistently failed to draw on the vast literature which has developed since the earliest times around the subject of aesthetics and the theory of art. We need to draw on such theories and insights in order to clarify and elaborate our own aesthetic vocabulary. (Holmes, 1991, p. 445)

It seems a little odd that he should speak of the theory of art rather than its practices here. But, he adds:

> In what sense is nursing an art? What right have we to insist that nursing *is* an art? To what does the word *art* refer here? How important in this context is the *process* of art as compared to the *product*? What epistemological or ontological status has *aesthetic knowledge*, and is it to be identified with that derived from the apprehension of a work of art? Ought we to characterize expert nursing as a *craft*, and if we do, is that different to saying it is an art, or is craft a category of art? Where do *artistry and skill* fit into the picture? Is all therapeutic nursing a form of art, and all artistic nursing therapeutic? . . . . How does this perspective help us to improve the quality of nursing care? (Holmes, 1991, p. 445–446)

Holmes asks important questions here, but then proceeds to become entangled in aesthetics (the philosophical questions about art, including whether art has a moral function). He asks questions about the relationship between art and intuition and pursues the notion of how art and craft are related and where skills lie in all this. However, Holmes does not look in detail either at art forms themselves or at specific nursing practice in order to try to see where the language he is using comes from, or how it relates to the real work of practitioners. But he does offer a review of work across aesthetic, anthropological and theatrical scholarship citing particularly Schechner and Appel (1990), which offer 'promising springboards from which to begin exploring the notion of nursing as aesthetic performance'. And he looks forward to the day when we have a 'theory of nursing aesthetics' to balance all those 'theories of nursing science' (Holmes, 1991, p. 451).

Holmes is certainly keen to develop our understanding about professional artistry in respect of nursing, and his ideas build broadly beyond what Carper offered earlier, but like her, and also like Schön to some extent, these are ideas about ideas. Holmes' work contributes to the questions rather than offering ways forward in understanding concrete examples. By contrast, the work of nurse educators offers a different and very important perspective because in Britain in the early 1990s the new Project 2000 courses for entry to nursing were being designed. Many professionals at this time were grappling with more practical questions about what to teach and how to teach trainee nurses.

Project 2000: the common curriculum and the art and craft of nursing

Keen and Shannon (1991) offer one usefully clear example of this. They start from the belief that 'the complexity of nursing rests not in the performance of manual skills but in communicating with people who are in pain, anxious, frightened and isolated' (Shannon, 1987, p. 3), and that this requires 'a curriculum framework which recognizes the primacy of the interpersonal and interactional nature of care'. They do not seek to undermine the technical aspects of nursing, but seek to see the development of the ability to make relationships as more important even than the nursing actions, role responsibilities and procedures, because the nurse/patient relationship is the context for all the rest. They therefore make the nursing interactions with patients the core of their curriculum and place the science of nursing and the art of nursing on either side of it, feeding into it. They offer the following five headings as their attempt at defining the art of nursing: courage, empathy, design, creativity and risk. But the scope of the article does not allow them to consider in detail whether these capacities and characteristics are really endemic to and definitive of *artistry*, or if they are merely qualities generally admired. As we shall now see, this has certainly also been a concern of other nursing literature of the 1990s.

An examination of the art of nursing

The issue of what is meant by expertise in nursing and why it should be seen as an art is explored by Hampton (1994) – but in ways that are not entirely helpful because she certainly seems to be using the term merely as a mark of quality or value, to indicate her approval. By contrast, Johnson's work is much more informative, drawing as it does on the work of forty-one American authors in order to 'discover the common ground that underlies the differences of opinion regarding the art of nursing and to transmute the current diversity into rational and intelligible controversy'. This involves formulating 'patterns of agreement and disagreement' (Johnson, 1994, pp. 1–2). She complains (quite rightly) that the term 'nursing art' is not well understood, that there is 'a plethora of diverse views concerning the art of nursing [which] are relatively unquestioned and unexplored' and that a 'state of fragmentation . . . characterizes the nursing literature relevant to the subject of nursing art'. She concludes that there are diverse answers to the question: What is the art of nursing? The use of the term 'art of nursing' in no way ensures that those involved in the discourse refer to the same subject. She does however find five separate 'senses' of nursing art, although she says that these are not mutually exclusive and several are usually found together in the writings. These are:

1   the nurse's ability to grasp meaning in patient encounters;
2   the nurse's ability to establish a meaningful connection with the patient;
3   the nurse's ability to skilfully perform nursing activities;
4   the nurse's ability to rationally determine an appropriate course of nursing action; and
5   the nurse's ability to morally conduct his or her nursing practice (Johnson, 1994, p. 3).

In the first of these the focus is on the uncertainty, ambiguity and indeterminacy that render the patient's situation and the nurse's role complex, and on the increase of this problem when patients are unable to be articulate about their needs. In these cases the artful nurse is one who can grasp what is significant in a particular patient situation. This involves the senses and the imagination, a recognition of the emotional as well as the cognitive. Nursing art involves the perceptual capacity, and often, intuition rather than reasoning or reflection. Here the abilities and capacities involve 'sensing the meaning', observing imaginatively, perceiving patterns, having a feel, 'knowing' when to do what. There is a strong sense in some of the literature that these abilities are exercised holistically. This is a form of understanding that defies accurate description because the insights are tacit, but it can be learnt with experience. (And although Johnson does not say so, it can be communicated and shared by artistic means.) (See Johnson, 1994, pp. 4–5.)

The second of these involves 'bridging the gap left by technology'. It emphasizes 'wholeness and integrity in the personal encounter'. Here, making connections is important. Also, it is non-discursive (it is in the doing rather than in discussion) and is 'unmediated by conceptual categories'. It is 'an experience lived between human beings' and 'involves the expression of the nurse's state of being'. It also demands authenticity on the part of the nurse. 'The artful nurse must be genuine' because anything else will distance nurse from patient (see Johnson, 1994, pp. 5–7).

The third of these is about skilful performance (manual and verbal). The artful nurse 'knows more than what is to be done, she knows how to do it'. Here nursing is a behavioural activity. Heidgerken's useful words are quoted: 'the principles, procedures and technics, or science, of nursing are learnt in the classroom. The skill or art of nursing is learnt on the ward'. Benner and Wrubel argue that nurses' actions are effective when they have a sophisticated repertoire of reactions (see Johnson, 1994, pp. 7–8).

The fourth category involves the rational and practical abilities of nurses. Again nursing art is 'action oriented' and there is an underlying discipline of problem-solving. Here an artful nurse thinks 'logically, soundly and searchingly', and nurses' actions are not automatic but grounded in intellectual ability (see Johnson, 1994, pp. 8–10).

The final category links art to ethics. 'A nurse may be technically competent and knowledgeable, yet if he or she does not make moral choices in the performance of patient care, he or she is not artful' (see Johnson, 1994, pp. 10–12).

Johnson concludes that few authors acknowledge others' conceptions and even that there has been little recognition that differences exist. In offering categories which focus on art as well as aesthetics, the article provides a basis for future developments in defining what art in nursing is and how it should be pursued and developed. It should be remembered however that this article is American-based and charts territory much less well treated in Britain. Here the work of Carper was beginning to gain ground in the early 1990s.

Carper's work reviewed

In 1994, the journal *Advances in Nursing Science* recognized formally the pressure to consider the artistry of nursing, and, despite its title, set out bravely to explore these issues in an entire edition called *Esthetics and the Art of Nursing*. This in itself shows the prominence being given to artistry as the millennium approaches.

In the editorial to this issue, Chinn noted the seminal work of Carper and its enormous influence upon almost all studies on the art of nursing. She argued that Carper's work has stood the test of time and debate, and that although there are now 'equally viable interpretations concerning patterns of knowing that build on Carper's work', her real contribution has been in 'opening doors of possibility for nursing knowledge development' which led to 'widespread recognition that nurses and nursing depend on and need forms of knowing in addition to and other than empirics alone'. This is no doubt true. She says:

> In part because of the door that Carper opened, philosophical inquiry, particularly related to nursing ethics, has become a valued and valuable method of inquiring in nursing. Methods associated with art and esthetics, as with personal knowing, have been slower to evolve and develop. (Chinn, 1994, p. viii)

One wonders whether this might be because in some senses Carper set those who would pursue such matters in directions which took them away from the Arts, pointing as she did to the realm of aesthetics rather than art and perhaps causing other writers and thinkers to turn to epistemology and to start with theories rather than exploring specific art itself and starting with specific nursing practice.

Chinn adds rather more helpfully than almost anything Carper says about art:

> esthetic expression moves into levels of awareness and understanding that cannot be translated or explained in the more familiar approaches of empirical or philosophic inquiry. Despite this challenge, like the authors whose work appears in this issue, I have persisted in exploring esthetics, recognizing that deep meanings of human experience associated with health and illness defy expression in any medium other than what we know as art. (Chinn, 1994, p. viii)

In other words, through the Arts we can express the ineffable, the tacit, the responses and reactions to situations which are otherwise unable to be articulated but which are an important part of the complex symphony of human interaction which needs to be understood as a whole if practice is to be finely attuned to its particular context.

She also points out that aesthetic enquiry 'is beginning to raise interesting questions about what it means to know' and also proceeds, very helpfully, to categorize the directions, or dimensions in aesthetic knowing that are currently being pursued by thinkers and researchers. These are:

- the development of artistic expression by nurses to convey aesthetic meaning known through the experience of nursing;
- developing an understanding of nursing as an art form including how it is expressed and the inspiration from which it flows;
- the study of an artist's work to gain deep understanding of human experiences related to health and illness;
- the use of art as a therapeutic, healing or learning tool (see Chinn, 1994, p. viii).

It is the first two of these with which this book is mainly concerned. The third category (which was originally developed in the context of the education of doctors), though fascinating, is only tangential to the intentions of this book. It includes the work in medical humanities of Beckingham (1986), of Rowena Murray (see for example Robb and Murray, 1992) in nursing and of Thow and Murray (1991), which introduces this approach to physiotherapists). Medical humanities offer:

> an innovative way of learning. Discussing literary texts of nursing practice has been used to help students analyse attitudes, values and ethics; it has also been used to help practitioners review and reflect on their own experience and philosophy of nursing. In nursing education, it has been used to explore difficult issues in a safe environment. (Robb and Murray, 1992, p. 1182)

This category of Chinn's also includes other recent work in using literary studies to help doctors, nurses and others to gain insights into areas of human thought and feeling that are normally difficult to express: see, for example, work with nurses on compassion (Young-Mason, 1988); an article called 'Can poetry help us to become better psychiatrists?' (Holmes, 1996); and 'The use of Literary Classics in teaching medical ethics to physicians' (Radwany and Adelson, 1987). Examples of Chinn's fourth category are included in Part 3 of Chinn and Watson (1994) (which is considered below) but also extend to new uses of image-making in research and enquiry itself (see, for example, Spouse, 1994).

Clearly, then, Chinn's review of Carper's work is particularly helpful in categorizing approaches to considering the aesthetics of nursing practice. Chinn has done much to work towards the recognition and clarification of the artistry of practice. Her 1994 anthology of art and aesthetics in nursing (co-edited with Watson) is a remarkable and unique attempt to offer a major arena in which to examine the detail of the role of art in professional artistry, which can only be given brief treatment here.

Chinn and Watson's Art and Aesthetics in Nursing
In a special introduction to their anthology, Watson and Chinn set the tone for its more direct consideration of art. They say: 'art conspires with the spirit to emancipate us; art allows us to locate ourselves in another space and place, to change our perceptions, our points of view. The relations of the parts and the whole shift' (Watson and Chinn, 1994, p. xv). There follows a major collection of work in four sections: art as asking and knowing; art as learning; art as practice; and art as reflective experience. Of particular interest are the two chapters by Vezeau, one by Maeve and one by Breunig. Vezeau notes that 'the usual outcome of narrative is not certainty . . . but the discovery of salient questions . . . which were not envisioned prior to the narrative' (Vezeau, 1994a, p. 43). She also offers comments on the rigour and trustworthiness of narrative and declares that 'creative fiction has long been an underground pursuit amongst nurses' (Vezeau, 1994a, p. 61). She also notes that 'for all that has been written about aesthetic knowing, little work has been encouraged or published' until now (Vezeau, 1994b, p. 180). The work of Maeve is on the moral dimension of art. She offers a useful review of writers who have used narratives to explore morality, and argues that 'art has traditionally reflected the moral consciousness of the artist and has informed the moral consciousness of the spectator, observer or participant' (Maeve, 1994, p. 75). The work of Breunig is fascinating because she has been both a professional artist and a professional nurse. She describes as similar the creative thrust of her work in both fields. She says that as a painter she regularly tried to control all aspects of a painting:

> until they became like a million loose threads on a loom that was hell-bent on weaving itself. Then something very subtle would shift in me. I would give up trying to hold on to the reins . . . . there would be a timeless time. When I looked up some moments or hours later, there would be an image on the canvas that was not of my

own doing. There was a rightness about the forms and colors . . .
(Breunig, 1994, p. 192)

She adds:

> In the creative moment of an artist, there is a person, paint, and
> canvas. In the caring moment, there is a nurse, a client, and the
> circumstances of their lives. The tools are not brush and canvas;
> they are empathy, reflection, metaphor, reframing and caring.
> (Breunig, 1994, pp. 193–194)

This book is certainly unique. It is to be hoped that it will encourage further work in this field and open up publishing to writers
who may be holding back because they fear that what they have
to say is not 'academic' enough or because the spirit of the times
seems antithetical to them.

Meanwhile, Chinn's work in exploring these matters has continued further, picking up themes we met earlier and in rather more
traditional terms. Of this, Chinn and Kramer (1995) seems typical.

Aesthetics and the art of nursing: Chinn and Kramer 1995

Chinn and Kramer, in offering further ideas about nursing's patterns of knowing, draw attention to the fact that they use the term
intuition (as an aspect of aesthetic knowing) rather differently from
Carper. They argue that 'esthetic knowing in nursing is made visible through the actions, bearing, conduct, attitudes, and interactions of the nurse in response to others'. Esthetic knowing makes
it possible to know what to do instantly, without conscious deliberation (Chinn and Kramer, 1995, p. 10).

They add that 'esthetic knowing'

> involves the creative processes of engaging, intuiting, and envi-
> sioning . . . . The experience does not depend on mental structures
> or cognitive representations or explanations. Rather, the meaning
> of the moment comes from deep within the subjective experience, is
> intuited from the context of the individual's, human experiences and
> becomes expressed through in-the-moment being in the situation.
> Intuiting leads directly to creative responses to the unique meaning
> of the moment and envisioning of new creative possibilities. (Chinn
> and Kramer, 1995, p. 10)

Citing Benner (1984), and the work of Chinn discussed above, they
continue:

> Like personal knowing, esthetics is not expressed in language but artistically in the moment of experience–action. We refer in this text to the expression of the art/act, because nursing's art form tends to be the artful ways in which nurses interact with people and perform skilled tasks .... Each art/act is a unique and particular instance that cannot be replicated. (Chinn and Kramer, 1995, pp. 10–11)

They offer, as examples of 'esthetic knowing', comforting someone in pain. They say that certain traits of comforting such a person can be communicated, and the behaviours associated with comforting can be learnt, but the esthetic knowing involved is 'expressed directly in the art/act; it only occurs in the moment and is unique to the particular esthetic experience. What is shared in the art/act becomes part of shared understanding in the discipline'. But how is it shared when there seems to be no common language for it? This is indeed where art could help.

Chinn and Kramer add, coming perhaps closest to the thrust of the arguments in my Chapters 6 and 7, that criticism and consensus are the processes that contribute to forming understanding in aesthetics, because criticism (as in art criticism) reveals meanings, creates insights, and provides interpretations that help others to appreciate more fully what the artist has done. They argue that it 'can move beyond what is, to something that might be in the future'. They define criticism as 'deliberate, critical, precise, thoughtful reflection and action directed toward transformation' (Chinn and Kramer, 1995, p. 11–13).

A summary of issues in the artistry of nursing: the 1980s and the 1990s
The 1980s then were dominated, in the (mainly North American) literature cited, by considering aesthetics as a way of knowing in nursing, and by a focus on intuition. It was clear even at this stage that one of the main problems was going to be finding a language in which to express some of these ineffable ideas, and that there was a temptation either to avoid the detail by dismissing much of it as common sense or to brand intuition in barely disguised technical rational terms as 'a sophisticated form of reasoning'. By comparison, some writing in the 1990s has attempted to come to grips with the detail of art and artistry in nursing practice and less with aesthetics as such, but that even here, with the distinguished excep-

tion of the work of Chinn, the advances in understanding artistry have been slow to emerge.

If Carper influenced the nursing literature on art and artistry, on both sides of the Atlantic, it was Schön who influenced it in physiotherapy and occupational therapy, where his notions about reflection have been picked up, but his ideas about artistry have not.

Artistry in occupational therapy and physiotherapy

There is much less in the literature on occupational therapy and physiotherapy about the artistry of practice. This is perhaps because of the paramount need which has long been felt in both professions to establish 'solid knowledge' (scientific knowledge) as an important basis of their claim to professional status as well as because both professions are much smaller than nursing. For occupational therapy the term 'art' still has associations perhaps with the therapeutic skills they teach their patients. For physiotherapy the vital knowledge base is regarded traditionally as science itself, which is seen as central to professional understanding. As Sim notes: physiotherapists 'are educated in a predominantly biomedical context' (Sim, 1990, p. 427). But beneath the surface of this, many issues arise in practice that demonstrate the need for and indeed the use of more artistic perspectives. However, in many cases such characteristics are not *referred to* as art. This seems to be either because they are not recognized as such, or because reference to art is consciously – or subconsciously – seen as unhelpful to their image.

Nevertheless, signs of growing awareness of the need for more than a science base to physiotherapy are emerging amongst practitioners, and researchers who believe in the primacy of practice (believe in researching practice and practitioners) and who write for the professional audience. For example, Beeston and Simons (1996) show how an examination of a sample of physiotherapist *practitioners'* perspectives reveals that they see their work as far more than simply scientific. Indeed, although they do not mention the word art, they provide many examples of and comments about practice by physiotherapist practitioners which echo what we have already found in the nursing literature.

Beeston and Simons' article draws upon semi-structured interviews with a sample of physiotherapists who had been in practice for between five and thirty-three years and who had worked in Greater London in a variety of settings within which neurophysiotherapy was carried out. A picture emerged of 'patient-centred values, practice-centred knowledge and profession-specific action' (Beeston and Simons, 1996, p. 238). They found that physiotherapists first gained an overall picture of the patient and only then focused upon patients' ability to move. (Here we have again the importance of the holistic view which, as we shall see in Chapters 6 and 7, is a central idea in the Arts and in the appreciation of the Arts.) Using a metaphor from the Arts, Beeston and Simons add that physiotherapists concentrated on what they as writers characterize as 'working in harmony with the patient and the carer' (Beeston and Simons, 1996, p. 236). (Again, harmony is a major focus of interest in the arts.) They report too that:

> Harmony was seen in the interplay between mobilizing and facilitating, in the way in which patients 'recognize' and 'feel' the movements which they are unable to perform alone, and where physical handling by the therapist involves patient co-operation and carryover [sic].
> In the view of the respondents, such harmony in the physical realm needed to be accompanied by an equal commitment to the psychological aspects of care. (Beeston and Simons, 1996, p. 237)

The writers observe later that working in harmony 'is a strongly collaborative model', but there is no scope for them to pursue this. Their respondents mostly argued that theoretical knowledge was only valued if it could 'answer the complex and practical problems encountered within practice'. They added that 'feel' was 'an important factor for the therapist', that knowledge about 'handling' a patient (literally) was 'a part of the tacit knowledge of the expert practitioner', and that 'the quality of empathy and the need for it were very evident' (Beeston and Simons, 1996, pp. 240–241). They reported that:

> most [practitioners] now described themselves as eclectic and were reluctant to identify with any one approach. Their starting point was the needs of individual patients. Their practice was not premised on research findings or on any one theory. (Beeston and Simons, 1996, p. 241)

They further noted that 'this was not an area of practice where it was possible for practitioners to use treatment protocols'. This is clearly then an article which seeks to pave the way for further work in this field, and which in acknowledging the need for this, demonstrates the 'state of the art' of thinking about artistry in physiotherapy.

By contrast to physiotherapy, occupational therapy has not turned to pure science to establish its credentials but has struggled much more to define its knowledge base. When challenged, the profession (rather ironically) tends to emphasize a humanistic approach to health care by turning to (or creating) theoretical models (see Adamson *et al.*, 1994; Hagadorn, 1995; Kielhofner, 1995). None of these mentions art, nor does the influential American work of Mattingly and Fleming (1994). But Hagadorn (1997) begins to chart this territory and use new language.

It is Rogers though who articulates on behalf of occupational therapy a view of artistry which also sounds very similar to views offered in the nursing literature. Almost echoing Carper (whom she does not cite in her bibliography), she says the clinician 'functions as a scientist, ethicist and artist' and adds that these dimensions are inextricably intertwined. She declares that 'Artistry involves the orchestration of broad strategies for grappling effectively with the uncertainties inherent in clinical practice' (Rogers, 1983, p. 614). Referring to Schön, she adds that artistry 'is revealed in our actions . . . in knowing what to do and how to do it'. She then actually turns to the Arts for help and utilizes analogies from music to help her explain further what is involved in the work of an occupational therapist. She says 'we get a feel for the skill and that feeling allows us to repeat our performance'. She continues:

> know how to touch the piano keys to play a Mozart piano concerto, and your artistry is apparent in your music. If you were to describe your 'knowing how to play' the piano, you would find this difficult . . . . Clinical reasoning may be viewed as a skill akin to piano playing. The skill consists of reducing the ambiguities inherent in clinical practice to manageable risks, and by so doing enabling the formulation of prudent decisions. (Rogers, 1983, p. 614)

For Rogers this process involves the very kinds of skills named by Johnson above (interpersonal skills, building trust, explaining alternatives to patients, offering encouragement, gathering cues adeptly, probing for information not volunteered, clarifying discrepancies, recognizing patterns, perceptual acuity, thinking on one's feet). Here then, we have a writer from occupational therapy couching her exploration of the artistry of her profession in the language of the Arts rather than aesthetics.

Artistry and Traditional Chinese Medicine

I have neither the knowledge nor the skill to do justice to the views about professional artistry enshrined in Traditional Chinese Medicine – that is, the system of medicine which originated in China in antiquity and has formed the theoretical basis of the medical systems which developed in China and its neighbours, such as Japan, Korea, Taiwan and Vietnam (see Mole, 1992, p. 115). But it is clear even to a lay person that those therapeutic activities which rest upon Traditional Chinese Medicine, and which are currently undergoing considerable expansion in the West, take a similar view to those quoted above about matters to do with art and science, theory and practice, mind and body. But where Western medicine and its associated professions are only now returning to these views, Traditional Chinese Medicine has always avowedly seen the human being as an integral part of his or her environment and treated the patient 'as a whole rather than treating the symptoms out of context of the human being who has the symptoms'. Sickness is thus understood in Traditional Chinese Medicine as 'the dysfunction of a normally harmonious, complete living entity' rather than a small part of a 'sophisticated biochemical and mechanical machine' (Mole, 1992, p. 112). The mind and body are never considered as separate from each other and the spirit is also part of this whole. Balance and harmony together with a respect for the particularity of each individual are key concepts. 'While all systems of medicine can be practised more or less holistically . . . Chinese medicine places the diagnosis of the patient at the core of its diagnostic process' (see Mole, 1992, pp. 5–6). Even here we see in the use of words like 'harmony' and 'holistic' notions also common to art. And acupuncture as an example of a profession based upon Traditional Chinese Medicine accepts positively the dual aspects of science and art that are part of its character. For example, Mole says 'the science of acupuncture is based upon detailed observations of how people change when they become ill .... The art of acupuncture depends upon the sensitivity and intuition of the practitioner' (Mole, 1992, p. 113).

Issues in artistry from the health care professions

An overview of this literature then allows us to see some major patterns. There is more evidence of writers talking of the artistry of their profession and of their professions as (partly) involving art than there is of writers merely utilizing handy figures of speech to explain some detail of practice. There is little agreement on the characteristics of artistry in professional practice beyond the recognition of intuition, creativity and a beyond-the-book response to particular circumstances of practice. And there is still little consensus on a definition of artistry in practice even within one profession. What does emerge, however, is a strong sense that there is much that happens in professional practice in health care that could be better discussed, explored and shared if only its artistic nature were more clearly articulated and professionals were equipped with the language and ideas in which the Arts themselves are discussed. There is a clear sense here, then, that in much of this writing the notion of professional artistry is indeed a vision rather than a mirage and has some substance, even if the vision is a little blurred.

By comparison, the literature on teaching and teacher education attends in less detail to intuition, but does utilize language and ideas directly from the Arts to look at some details of teaching. In it we can see the benefits of confronting centrally the question: In what sense is teaching an art? And we can see from that confrontation that this idea is far from being a mere mirage.

Teaching as a paradigm case of artistry

Teaching, like nursing, offers much literature which tackles the subject of professional artistry. The following collects together a few outstanding examples.

Teachers are artists: the work of Lawrence Stenhouse

The work of Stenhouse, written in the late 1970s at a time of some stability in British education, represents a direct attempt at portraying teaching *as* artistry. Where others speak of the artistry to be found in practice, here Stenhouse (developing a persuasive metaphor) makes an unequivocal statement about a teacher *being* an artist. He emphasizes the importance of seeing action and idea holistically in teaching activities (and this is akin to the important unity of form and content that, in the classic definition makes for good art in all the Arts). In indicating that the teacher works to become an individual artist by going beyond previous examples of the tradition of (teaching) practice, he strikes a familiar chord for teacher readers, provides a further important insight for those seeking to understand their teaching better, and introduces ideas which Eisner later extends.

Teachers are like artists: the ideas of Eliot Eisner

Eisner's early attempts at working on the artistry in teaching are to be found in the article published in 1983, some details from which were presented and discussed in Chapter 2.

Clearly, although its motives are understandable and he properly calls attention to it by switching in and out of artistic imagery, the article is propaganda (of a kind we could currently well do with). For example, the reader is deliberately swept along by the speed of the rhetorical cadences created by his short closed questions followed by brief assertive answers. And yet it could be argued that this display of virtuosity instead of detracting from the argument about the power and use of artistic imagery as a means of understanding teaching, actually illustrates it. Eisner writes unequivocally, and, as we saw in Chapter 2, he does seem to have identified aspects of the teacher's role which can legitimately be described as artistry and in so doing he does enable us to identify and to focus on aspects of teaching that currently are often overlooked, hard to capture, and difficult to describe in the more precise language of technical rationality. Later he was to extend this theme in his well-known book *The Art of Educational Evaluation* (1985), where he turned to the idea of the appreciation of the artistry of the teacher. But we shall look at this in more detail in Chapter 6.

Using art to explore teaching: some recent examples

In addition to exploring notions of teaching as artistry there is a huge literature which uses ideas from the Arts to understand aspects of the complex processes involved in the practice of teaching and the processes of learning to practise. See particularly the work of Richard Winter (Winter, 1986, 1988; and also Landgrebe and Winter, 1994, which extends this work into the health field, and Rowland, Rowland and Winter, 1990). He explores the value of fictional writing and narrative as 'a way of coming to terms with experience and as providing confidence with which to challenge unaccepted theories and encourage agendas for further learning' (Landgrebe and Winter, 1994, p. 83: see also the entire issue of *Educational Theory*, 1995, volume 45, number 1). The literature on the use of narrative in professional research and development is also huge (see for example, Connelly and Clandinin, 1986, 1990, 1995; Egan, 1988; Gudmundsdotter, 1991; Jalongo, 1992; Tripp, 1993; Weber, 1993; see also the work of Groundwater-Smith, 1984, p. 1, who looks at literary non-fiction which can portray 'factual information as a complex counterpointing of description and explanation', and Schostak, 1985, on the processes involved in such writing). The work of Munby (1986) and Chinn (1994, p. 4) on metaphor is also of considerable interest. The other major literature is in learning to teach, and much of this struggles to make artistry explicit. Two examples must suffice. Both draw upon music and are interconnected.

In an interesting article which looks at processes of learning to teach involving a student, a teacher and a college lecturer – or triad as it is commonly dubbed – Gore seeks to encourage staff to practise what they themselves preach in terms of reflection on practice and their personal investigation of their own practice. In preparing to investigate her own work in a triad she clarifies the notion of the triad by saying: 'The term itself simply implies a group of three closely related persons or things, or, in music, a chord of three tones' (see Gore, 1991, p. 154).

Later she talks of two different symbols to describe the threesome – a triangle and a triad – and notes how 'the choice of symbols . . . has implications for the way we think about and conduct our work' (Gore, 1991, p. 267). She notes that the dissonance between these two possible symbols for the teaching triad gave the focus to her own research project. She then pursues a greater understanding of the relationships within the triad through musical analogy.

> In music a triad is a chord made up of a root [the key note] and its third and fifth. Who is the root in the student teaching triad? One might assume that it is the student teacher but . . . it seems that the supervisor plays a major role in establishing the triad . . .
>
> On the other hand, perhaps it *is* appropriate to talk of the student teacher as the root; in music, the root gives the central focus to the tonality. The supervisor might then be considered the third; in music the third is perhaps the most important note because it determines whether it is a major or minor triad. Perhaps the supervisor determines how the triad functions while the student provides the . . . *raison d'être*. But what of the co-operating teacher? (Gore, 1991, p. 267)

She goes on to note that:

> the symbol triad implies harmony, 'a pleasing or congruent arrangement of parts', musical notes in a harmonious chord . . . . An unsuccessful triad is characterized as dissonant, a clashing musical interval, an unresolved musical chord, a lack of agreement. (Gore, 1991, p. 268)

She might have added that music needs these too in order to develop and explore its original themes, but she does say that dissonance may be necessary for learning to occur. She concludes by saying that whilst she does not want to push these ideas too far, 'there is some value in thinking of the student teaching triad as chamber music' (Gore, 1991, p. 268).

These ideas are explored further by Peterat and Smith, who offer reflections 'illuminated metaphorically through considering the student teaching triad as chamber music' (Peterat and Smith, 1996, p. 15). They make the point in their abstract that 'the music metaphor enables an account of the resonances and dissonances; the frustrations, doubts and discomforts within collaborative projects', and certainly allows them to explore collaboration itself. They also use the word 'refrain' (a phrase or verse repeated regularly in a song or a poem) saying that 'the refrains occurring in the student teaching practicum are often called by others "dilemmas" or "problems"' (Peterat and Smith, 1996, p. 21). And they attempt to illustrate issues about improvising which they define as 'composing on the spur of the moment'.

It is an interesting question as to whether all this work is entirely successful and totally persuasive. Careful distinctions perhaps need to be drawn between metaphors, analogies and symbols which genuinely foster new thinking about practice, and the invention of such figures for their own sake or merely to refresh stale ideas. None the less, these are examples of the felt need to express professional practice in artistic terms and thereby to understand it better.

Conclusions

Thus we have established that many professions use the term artistry fairly extensively in discussing professional practice and that there is no one simple definition of it. We have also noted that in some cases professional practice is described as *like* or *similar to* activities in painting, literature, drama or music, and that in other cases it is described *as* such an Art. It is also clear that there are common threads running through the various definitions and discussions cited above. Professional artistry is about practical know-how, skilful performance or knowing-as-doing, and is not easy to express in verbal form – not simply because it is tacit knowledge which practitioners have failed to make explicit even for themselves, but because it is by its very nature non-verbal. Professional artistry seems to be characterized by the following:

- intuition
- creativity – inventing new moves, taking calculated risks, making new practice on the spot in practice
- improvisation
- imagination
- going beyond the rules, and the rule book
- seeing one's practice in relation to the traditions and conventions of the work of one's profession
- operating through trial and error, taking chances, going beyond the known
- displaying overall competence in uncertain situations
- the ability and capacity to make professional judgements in difficult circumstances

- being concerned with the holistic nature of the situation, with seeing the overall picture, attending to patterns
- the ability to see ahead from within a situation – to 'envision' how things will be in the future
- having a feel for a situation, being able to empathize with those involved, and being good at recognizing expressive nuance
- thinking critically, being self-critical and being willing to 're-write' and re-think
- using on-the-spot experimentation
- recognizing and responding to unique phenomena
- theorizing in and from the situation
- learning from and within the practical situation
- framing problems with artistry in mind
- doing many things at once
- thinking on one's feet, feeling one's way through the situation.

In the light of all this, it seems clear that the notion of professional artistry is indeed a vision rather than a mirage.

In asking why such issues matter in our technological and scientific world we have argued that the notion of professional artistry enables us to defend the very character and significance of professionalism itself. This is because professional work that was able totally to be regulated by procedures decided beforehand and outside the situation would be both dangerous to the public (because life is not like that) and inimical to professionalism (because it would down-grade professionals, making them servants of bureaucracy and mere sub-professionals). We have thus also concluded that the use of the term 'artistry' is more than a means of indicating that practice is generally valued. Rather it offers useful ways of understanding it better. All this shows that being more articulate about the artistry in our practice is a vital means of explaining and defending our professionalism.

How then can we explore the artistry of practice? What conditions might help us to investigate and write about it appropriately?

4

Practitioner as artist: professional development through critical appreciation

Introduction

The words of Stenhouse, used originally to characterize teaching and rephrased to include health care, seem the most appropriate beginning to a chapter on professional development. He wrote:

> [Professional practitioners] must be educated to develop their art, not to master it, for the claim to mastery merely signals the abandoning of aspiration. [Professional practice] is not to be regarded as a static accomplishment like riding a bicycle or keeping a ledger; it is, like all arts of high ambition, a strategy in the face of an impossible task. (Stenhouse, in Rudduck and Hopkins, 1985, p. 124)

How then should professionals both learn their practice and continue to refine and develop it? On what basis can continuing professional development be established? These are perennial problems in the caring professions. Responses to them are shaped by differing beliefs and assumptions about how professionals work, think and learn and the differing values endemic to such ideas. This chapter will offer a response to these issues by providing first an overview of the arguments and then expanding on some details. For the purposes of this chapter, 'professional development' is taken to mean 'professional education', that is, *both* the initial preparation which develops students into professionals as well as the continuing professional development which is a career-long process. Indeed, there are strong arguments for seeing professional development as a seamless process.

An overview of the arguments presented here

As has been shown elsewhere, pre-registration health care (Coles, 1996), and initial teacher education courses (Fish, 1989, 1995a) take relatively little account of how professionals work, think and learn (Coles, 1996; Eraut, 1994). And this malaise has also affected the way continuing professional development is currently seen in many professions.

Because of the need for practitioners to keep up to date and to extend their expertise, most professions have over the years developed bureaucratic systems of professional development and incentives for working practitioners to take part in them. Striking examples of this have been seen in Continuing Medical Education in the 1990s (see Brigley *et al.*, 1996) and in occupational therapy in the 1980s. This kind of system has often enabled managers who wished to introduce (impose) changes, to use 'professional develop-ment' to engage outsiders to 'bring in' new knowledge with which to train professionals. The assumption here is that professional work is essentially technical rational and that only the TR aspects matter.

But, as we have seen in Chapter 3, many practitioners across all professions now claim that professional work involves working as an artist. This is because the practitioner is someone who, in a very real sense, is daily involved in meaning-making within practical situations which always have a moral dimension and a human face, who wrestles with complex and important thought and action, and who has to make complex professional judgements for which there can be no simple formula. Professionals also work with some inef-fable aspects of practice which are beyond anyone's ability to express in simple technical terms. And we know that all this activ-ity and thought is powerfully driven and shaped by the individual's beliefs and theories, assumptions and values that underlie his or her visible actions (see Fish and Coles, 1998).

Given such a view of what is involved in professional work, and since professional practitioners are like (or even are) artists, their developmental needs would seem likely to be similar to those experienced by poets, painters and musicians. This raises the question: how does an *artist* develop his or her art? Broadly, artists harness the processes of the critical appreciation of practice to gain insight into their own art and that of others in the same field.

What, then, is involved in critical appreciation? By critical appreciation is meant seeking to recognize the qualities of the work under scrutiny, attempting to respond appropriately to it as a whole, taking account of the context, the traditions and the conventions within which it was created, and discerning what is of significance in it for others. In this view, an artist develops his or her art by responding to and exploring his or her own and others' work with a view to understanding it better and thinking critically about it and how it relates to other practice extant within the tradition and field in which he or she practises. Critical appreciation is about the development of discernment. It takes an investigative approach to practice. It leads to lively and relevant debates and engages artists in (motivates them to) the simultaneous investigation of and development of both practice and theory, without the need for outside regulation and requirement.

The greatest irony of all here is that were anyone to seek to *impose* on any field of the Arts from the outside a prescription of what must count as 'quality' in that art, every thinking member of the public would realize how ridiculous, philistine and destructive that would be, and would see *inescapably* the damage it would do to the development of real quality in art. Working at clarifying the qualities that make something 'art' is precisely what *creating* art is all about, both for individual artists and for the world of the Arts, and it cannot be done by those who are outside that world. In many respects this is (and should also be recognized as) true of professional practitioners. Clearly professional practice has responsibilities to the public that artists do not have. But these are about being accountable, and thus about being able to give an account of one's practice. Critical appreciation is arguably, then, one of the best forms of accountability. Indeed, it is probably our previous inability to articulate these matters that has caught us up into our current state of siege.

One key, then, to establishing, developing and changing professional practice is for practitioners to utilize critical appreciation to understand better their own practice and that of others. This means concomitantly practising and investigating examples or incidents of that practice (seeing them holistically), preferably with the help of those experienced in such matters. In this sense, then, professional development is the same as that form of practitioner research which involves professionals investigating their practice. (This is sometimes referred to as 'insider practitioner research' to distinguish it from other kinds of research which is focused on practice but which does not engage practitioners in investigating their own work.) A key activity in both critical appreciation and insider practitioner research is for practitioners to bring the personal professional knowledge embedded in their practice to the surface and (with the help of the wider perspectives of the writing and thinking of others) to consider it critically in the light of the context, the traditions and the conventions of their profession as a whole. Thus, they will learn to see their practice anew and – of course – to discuss and write about it and to read the work of others engaged in the same process. In respect of this, Fish and Coles (1998) coined the metaphor of an iceberg to indicate the extent and detail of that which lies beneath the surface of practice.

These arguments suggest the need for a revised curriculum for both pre- and post-registration professional education. Here, professionals themselves would work at articulating their practice and 'theorizing it' with the help of higher education, research and critical friends, and thus become developers rather than subjects and recipients of practice-focused research. Here, higher education and research become the means of supporting the development of *practice* in the professions, and professional practice becomes the prime source of knowledge about practice.

These are arguments, therefore, for the reconceptualization of professional development as an educational rather than an administrative or technical activity (which is what it has become in many professions as a result of proceduralization), and as a research activity. Such an approach to professional education is both relevant *and workable* for those at pre-registration and at post-registration stages – for those engaged in formal courses and those caught up in the heat of practice. This is because it relies on few resources and demands no more time than professionals currently put in. Indeed, as we have shown (Fish and Coles, 1998, p. 311), it is possible to use that time for professional development which at the moment is spent on bureaucratic matters which may alter surface activities but which neither educate practitioners nor change their understanding. Further, it has far-reaching implications for ways of establishing, maintaining and refining standards, for quality assurance, for accountability (and its handmaid, audit), and for validation and accreditation procedures.

The following now takes up five key matters in greater detail: the professional development of the artist; practice as the source of professional knowledge; the meaning of critical appreciation; the role of appreciation of practice in quality assurance; some resource implications.

The artist and professional development

Stenhouse long ago showed us that there are parallels between these ideas for professional development and the way that artists themselves develop and refine their practice. For professionals and artists alike their knowledge base is the kind of knowing endemic in doing. They work on, and with, practical knowledge which is learnt in practice. In explaining that a teacher works (in the classroom) in the same way as an artist, Stenhouse argued that: 'artists . . . learn through the critical practice of their art'. He adds:

> thus in art ideas are tested in form by practice. Exploration and interpretation lead to revision and adjustment of idea and of practice. If my words are inadequate, look at the sketchbook of a good artist, a play in rehearsal, a jazz quartet working together. That, I am arguing, is what good teaching is like. (Stenhouse in Ruddock and Hopkins, 1985, p. 97)

We have only to look at the personal writings of artists – like the letters of Van Gogh, or Ruskin's *The Lamp of Beauty*, the writing about their own work of poets like Hughes and Frost, and the critical appreciation of the work of others by poets like Coleridge and T. S. Eliot – to see this point. In all these sorts of writing, those who engage regularly in the practice of creating, think and write about the processes involved, seeking always to improve their own work by learning from the critical consideration of it and of the work of others. This would seem to be the main way in which artists learn (although of course we also know that some artists of the Renaissance were apprentices in the matter of colour mixing). If professionals are artists in professional practice it seems reasonable to claim that they too need to utilize critical appreciation. But this is not the kind of appreciation for appreciation's sake. It is neither self-congratulatory nor is it characterizable by the vulgar term 'navel gazing'. It is interested neither in self-glorification nor therapy though it does involve self-knowledge. It may involve celebrating good practice, but it is at least as interested in routine practice, and in learning from uncertainty and the problems of practice. The central intention is to study practice in order to develop understanding and thus to develop practice. As Stenhouse says:

> Note, however, that the process of developing the art of the artist is always associated with change in ideas and practice. An artist becomes stereotyped or derelict when he ceases to develop. There is no mastery, always aspiration. And the aspiration is about ideas – content, as well as about performance – execution of ideas.

He adds:

> thus the process of developing one's art as a teacher – or the art of teaching, which develops through individual artists – is a dialectic of idea and practice not to be separated from change. (Stenhouse in Ruddock and Hopkins, 1985, p. 97)

This 'dialectic' of idea and action lies at the heart of critical appreciation, as we shall now see.

Educating the artist through critical appreciation

Armstrong, in a very useful book on responding to painting, eloquently shows that appreciation is a demanding activity, but that what is learnt is likely to be both significant and enduring, and (unlike many theoretical studies) will ultimately drive the 'appreciator' back to practice. He says:

> The appreciation of painting is an activity, or process, which has resonance in life beyond the time we actually spend looking at particular works. This means that, in the end, a full appreciation of the value of art will involve transcending the role of mere spectator. Throughout this book the active participation of the spectator has been emphasized: the active spectator contains the embryonic artist. (Armstrong, 1996, p. 139)

Armstrong argues that this means:

> that one should proceed for oneself with the task of the 'translation' of experience [of paintings studied]. This 'translation' amounts to the piecing together of the different strands of experience: it is the business of self-knowledge. What has really mattered to me, and why did it matter? What has gripped my attention, and why did it affect me in that way? (p. 139)

This, he says, involves 'perceptiveness towards the details of experience and discernment of the underlying themes of experience'. He adds:

> The quality of our relation to pictures cannot finally be divorced from the seriousness of our self-examination and our attentiveness to experience outside the gallery and outside the studio. In the pursuit of an appreciation of painting we are led, finally, to transcend our fascination with art. We turn to the contemplation of what it was that originally moved the artists we care for: the pleasures and mysteries of ourselves and the world. (Armstrong, 1996, p. 140)

This is essentially about 'ways of seeing'. One of the achievements of an artist is to see the world differently, and to capture that seeing so that it can be shared with others. The person who seeks to appreciate critically what the artist has done, recognizes and shares the artist's achievements, can draw others' attention to them, and is changed by such new understanding. Of course the artist's vision does not actually change the world (only the canvas). But, a 'new way of seeing' points up comparisons – between how we perceive a particular view and how the particular artist perceives it, between how we see (more generally) and how an artist 'sees', and between how things apparently are and how they might be. And here is where 'seeing' can become 'vision' and is bound to have a moral dimension.

Thus, in appreciating a particular painting we learn to see other paintings and the world anew. It takes an eye educated in discernment, enlightened by a clear understanding of the activity of appreciation, to recognize a new (moral) vision. But anyone willing to attend to the details of a painting and the means of appreciating it is embarking on such education, is on the way to new visions. Indeed, Phenix argued that not only the artist but any person who seeks to understand a given art form cultivates a feeling for the 'basic qualities, possibilities, problems and limitations of the materials from which objects in that field are made'. He characterizes the successful artist in any field as someone 'who thinks well with the *characteristic materials* of that field' (the musical composer, thinking with sounds, the painter with pigments, the sculptor revealing 'his intuitions in metal, clay, or marble', the architect speaking 'volumes with wood, brick, stone, steel' (Phenix, 1964, pp. 154–155). He adds that becoming expert in the arts 'grows out of prolonged imaginative experimentation with material media in order to exploit most fully the expressive possibilities of the substances used' (Phenix, 1964, p. 155). But the materials used are not significant, only the manner in which they are organized – how they are 'put together in a patterned whole' is what matters (Phenix, 1964, p. 156). Further, the work of art expresses 'something more than the immediate perceptual effects'. Though of course what a person sees in a piece of art 'depends considerably on his previous experience'.

We have seen, then, that artists learn from studying their practice and that of others. The assumption that underlies this is that for artists, practice is their prime source of knowledge. This seems self-evident and unexceptionable when we talk of artists, perhaps because we recognize some important issues about artistic know-how. In fact, similar arguments hold good for the practice of those in the professions. Here, equally, practice is the prime source of practical knowledge, and practitioners are makers of meanings in human situations, their characteristic materials being not just words but all the other means by which they interact with their patient, clients, students and colleagues.

Practice as the prime source of professional knowledge

In a professional context it is impossible to discuss the nature of practical knowledge without also discussing its relationship to theoretical knowledge and touching on the role of theory. (This is because professional practice – unlike art – has traditionally been prepared for by studying *theory*.) Further, as in art, the moral dimension of professional practice is also a vital element. The following, therefore is an attempt to shed some light on this.

Theory, practice and professional knowledge

In the past it has been traditional to divide courses of preparation for professional practice into theoretical (or propositional, that is, factual) knowledge and practical (or procedural, that is, process) knowledge, and even to teach propositional knowledge in a college classroom and procedural knowledge in a clinical setting, with different staff supporting each. More recently, however, professionals have come closer to understanding the importance of the approaches discussed above in relation to art. We understand that 'theory' is not important for its own sake, but as enlightening practice. We also see it differently. We now recognize that it comprises concepts, frameworks, ideas and principles which may be used to interpret, explain or judge intentions, actions and experiences (Eraut, 1994, p. 60). That is, theory is not simply that factual, public and formal knowledge gained from books and lectures. We now see procedural knowledge (practical knowledge) as far more valuable, complex and significant than we used to. And we recognize that *professional* knowledge includes procedural knowledge, propositional knowledge, practical knowledge, tacit knowledge, as well as skills and know-how (see Eraut, 1994, p. 16). It also involves the ability to deliberate (to engage in practical reasoning) and to theorize (to interpret, explain, judge intentions, actions and experiences) (see Eraut, 1994, p. 60). And it involves an awareness of the moral dimensions of the decision-making we engage in. Here we have a more crystallized version of what also happens when the artist works.

As we saw in Chapters 2 and 3, the personal knowledge which we engage to help us in a practical situation is usually a mixture of some formal knowledge which has been learnt in a classroom and some know-how which is inherent in the actions we are carrying out or which we have gained in previous similar situations, and it includes much tacit knowledge which we never bring to the surface, as well as theories we say we work to (espoused theories) and theories that really direct our simultaneous thinking and doing (theories-in-use) (see Eraut, 1994, pp. 16–18).

We argued in Fish and Coles (1998) that it is important for practitioners to recognize that theory underpins their practice, that they are theorists, that they can or should work at theorizing their practice, and that the moral dimension of their practice is what makes them professional. We agreed with Eraut that formal knowledge (theoretical knowledge formulated outside practice) cannot be directly applied in practice, but rather must be *transformed* by the practitioner if it is to be incorporated into the practitioner's personal knowledge and inform practice. Or, put another way, ideas become re-interpreted during use and may need to be used before they can be meaningful to the user. To achieve this there must be an ability and a willingness to theorize practice in response to the specific situation encountered. In a very real sense, then, professionals *create* professional knowledge (a mixture of personal theory and practical knowledge) *in* their practice (Eraut 1994, p. 43). Informal or personal theory is thus an invisible element of practice, and as such is often either overlooked or left as tacit in practitioners' accounts of their practice, as are many other important elements. Indeed, in Fish and Coles (1998) we used the image of an iceberg to help us represent many of the invisible elements of practice (Figure 4.1).

Although 'practical knowledge is expressed only in practice and learned only through experience with practice' (Eraut, 1994, p. 42), this does not mean in professional practice, any more than it does in the Arts, that practising is *all* that is involved. There also need to be ways of understanding that practice by means of reflection and investigation (which key processes are associated with critical appreciation). Neither does it mean that all practice is automatically good to follow and adopt. The taken-for-granted will always need to be challenged. A critical perspective and careful deliberation, brought to bear upon practice by the educated professional who has also considered the moral and ethical issues raised by professional practice generally, helps in determining what should be extended and what should be dropped. And this process is itself theorizing.

The primacy of practice

We noted in Fish and Coles (1998, pp. 19–22), that much of the human understanding (as opposed to content knowledge) that professionals need to draw upon during their working practice has until very recently simply not been developed in them during the

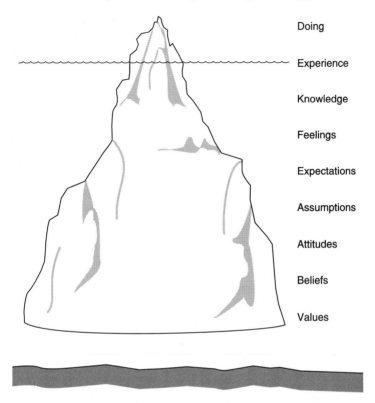

Doing

Experience

Knowledge

Feelings

Expectations

Assumptions

Attitudes

Beliefs

Values

Figure 4.1 The iceberg of professional practice

traditional course of professional preparation – and we pointed to making professional judgements as one major example of this. Instead, as we showed, formal theory and specialist knowledge have been and often still are emphasized during the taught course, and these are then treated as the basis for professional development and research. Students of such courses are thus left with the impression that practice only really gains its significance in an applicatory relationship to Formal Theory, and that it is (only) this formal theory that they should attempt to master and continue to develop during their working lives. But in fact, practical knowledge is a mixture of theorizing (being able to generate your own theory) and practising, and it is this which guides practice and needs continued development throughout a professional's career. (Hagar (1997, p. 115) argues that professional knowledge is an integral part of our practice.) This is why, once professionals begin work, their course of preparation to join their profession is often shown up as providing an inadequate basis for practice. For this reason, arguably, such courses should place major emphasis on practice, drawing personal theory out of practice and formal theory up to practice.

Thus, practice rather than theory is of prime significance for the professional practitioner – just as it is for the working artist. Practice is a reference point. It enables us both to give meaning to our ideas as they emerge from practice and to set the ideas which interest us back into context. Hagar quotes Cervero (1992) as making the point that 'a model of learning from practice should become a centrepiece of systems of continuing education for the professions' (see Hagar, 1997, p. 115). (Through such learning, of course, artists develop their work too.) Further, acquiring the capacity to ask increasingly complex and sophisticated evaluative questions about practice, and to investigate responses to these, is certainly a familiar activity for artists and could provide a useful agenda for professional development as a whole (see D. Carr, 1995, p. 323).

Individual practice and the practice of a profession

The term 'professional practice' can refer to the *individual activity* (or activities) of a single practitioner, but, equally, it can also refer to what Golby has called the 'whole tradition in which particular activities are related together as part of a social project or mission' (Golby, 1993, p. 4) – that is, to the practice of the whole profession itself. Indeed, the individual activities of a professional's practice, as Golby (1981) points out (or the individual work of an artist), needs to be understood from within the overall tradition of the practice of that profession (or of art) to which they belong. In this way the particular nature of the individual practice event can be appreciated both for its individual qualities and for the ways in which it relates to the traditions of practice more generally.

Thus, learning to become a professional (which continues throughout a professional's career) is 'a matter of coming ever more fully into membership of a tradition of practice' and, 'at its maturity it is a matter of taking part in more fully shaping practice for the future'. This involves understanding the inherited traditions of a profession (and/or of the preparation to enter that profession), and considering critically and practically their present relevance (see Golby, 1993, p. 8; Fish, 1995a, pp. 73–74; Fish and Coles, 1998, pp. 59–60). Equally, learning to understand the practice of an individual (or an individual artistic artefact) is at least partly a matter of coming to understand the traditions of that practice.

Professional know-how and know-how in the Arts: a summary

How similar then is professional know-how to know-how in the Arts? In both cases the know-how is inherent in the action itself – in the creation, in practice, of practical knowledge (which subsumes theory). In both cases practice is untidy and involves planning, problem-solving, analysing, evaluating, decision-making and a unique combination of propositional knowledge, situational knowledge and professional judgement. For both, there is no correct answer, no guaranteed road to success, only uncertainty about outcomes, a continual redefining of priorities, endless adjustment of propositional and procedural knowledge. In both cases self-knowledge is intrinsic to the processes. In both cases the guidance from theory is only partial; there is always insufficient contextual knowledge. There is in both cases a tension between previous custom and the immediate need to create new knowledge in situ. In both cases critics can illuminate the knowledge embedded in the processes and products of practice, but they cannot fully represent it in words. In both cases, normally, tacit knowledge needs to be articulated and subjected to critical scrutiny in order for practice to be developed. This involves practical reasoning. In both cases improving and refining practice can usefully be based upon learning to ask ever-increasingly sophisticated questions about practice, and in seeking ways to respond to them. Both involve moral responsibilities and require help in the development of fine judgement entailing moral and practical wisdom.

But there are also some significant differences. For example, in the case of many of the Arts, operating practical knowledge is a rather more solitary and meditative process than it is for professional practice, and there is not always an opportunity to consult others.

Given the extent of these similarities, and the arguments for both art and professional practice to be developed via critical appreciation, what exactly is this process?

The term critical appreciation

Professional practice is a highly complex activity which can be considered from a number of points of view. Some would argue that it can be analysed into its components. Some argue it can only be interpreted. Some, who argue for appreciation of such practice, maintain that it cannot really be fully atomized into separate components and deserves more than to be interpreted in one light. They seek to understand it more holistically.

Critical appreciation, then, is a process in which an activity or an object is responded to critically in order to understand it by any and as many means as possible, but which accepts that there may always be more means to understanding it than have been operated. This process seeks to consider the activity or object from many points of view, balancing pros and cons, seeking to set it in a context that helps to make sense of it, seeing in it meanings beyond the surface and seeing it as representative of something beyond it. This process involves the development of a discerning eye and the cultivation of sensitivities in relation to the objects appreciated. It sometimes seems that Marxism has appropriated the term 'critical', since that ideology seems to lie behind the term whenever it is mentioned. But such a 'critique' does not have to be Marxist if it is not couched in and shaped by terminology and ideas from that particular ideology. However, all critical appreciation is shaped by *some* beliefs and theories and it is important to indicate these as part of the critical response. The critical appreciation of an artistic artefact or a process (like professional practice) can (but need not) lead the 'appreciator' away from the activity or object under review towards larger matters.

It is possible to appreciate one's own practice, as well as that of others, both by reading about theirs and witnessing it. Critical appreciation reveals meaning, creates insights, provides interpretations, helps others to recognize what the artist has done. It teaches the critic to read situations without importing his or her own preconceptions, to recognize patterns, clarify discrepancies. It involves investigating, understanding, explaining. It reveals intuition, invention, insight. Placing the object or process within its context, identifying the traditions and conventions to which it relates in some way, enables one to offer a critique of the object or process and those very conventions and traditions which have shaped it. This leads to new and growing traditions, or new directions.

Like art and professional practice, critical appreciation – what Eisner (1985) calls connoisseurship – is a complex process, and further details of what is involved are to be found in Parts Two and Three where that practice is itself the key focus. It now remains, therefore, to consider the final two issues: the relationship of critical appreciation to quality assurance, and the resource implications of devoting professional development extensively to critical appreciation under the overall heading of insider practitioner research.

Critical appreciation and the re-focusing of quality assurance

It has been argued that quality in art clearly cannot be imposed from outside the art world, and that this is not about 'protecting the professional autonomy of artists' but about the nature of art as an activity. The same arguments apply to the world of professional practice. Only practitioners (of course with an ear to their clients' views) can establish and maintain the quality of their work. And the control of this quality across professional practice and across professions can only really be achieved from within the professional practice world. This is about self-study and self-regulation. Attempts at establishing standards from outside together with the inevitable inspection and control system which then must accompany it, *are inevitably a facade*, however much they are dressed up to appear otherwise. That is, they are bound to conduce to untruth and superficial changes, where self-study using critical appreciation within an insider practitioner research approach strains towards an honest appraisal of a situation and genuine attempts at improvement which run deep into personal knowledge. For this reason, accountability, and all its processes and handmaidens, need to be refocused. They need to be seen not as measuring individuals against a standard (never as objective or as useful as it would seem), but as enabling the individual to take responsibility for their own appraisal and improvement.

Indeed, it should be noted that those who embark upon activities like appraisal, audit and inspection (which lead to passing judgement upon the practice of professionals), and who take no account of the professional artistry endemic to that practice but work only on the basis of a technical rational view of professionalism and a technical rational exploration of that practice, are responsible for distorting our understanding in the short term and are in dire danger of having such judgements rebound upon them in the longer term.

Critical appreciation and insider practitioner research are a key means of establishing and ensuring quality in professional practice. They will enable professionals to reclaim their professionalism, to raise their moral awareness and to be articulate about their tacit knowledge (lack of which latter ability has made them an easy target of criticism in the past). Because it requires an acknowledgement of context, traditions, conventions, critical appreciation enables practitioners to refine their practice within the broad context of its value to society and develop (regain) their professional identity. And the cost of establishing this approach to professional development and accountability will be much less in resource terms than present systems.

Some resource implications

Time is one of the most important resources here. However, as will be clear from Part Three, insider practitioner research using critical appreciation does not require vast resources for generating or collecting and processing data or for travel to do so. It involves *inter alia* the production of a portrait of practice together with the investigation of that portrait and the practice, and the presentation of a critical commentary upon both. It certainly needs library resources, but all extended professionals (Hoyle, 1974) need such resources as a matter of course. It needs personnel to support it but again such people are either already in the professional's practice setting (and can easily become 'critical friends' to help in the appreciation, as we shall see below), or they are already involved in professional development.

Neither does it require more time than that already spent on professional work by the practitioner, but rather the redeployment of existing time. For example, as we noted in Fish and Coles (1998, p. 311), during the undergraduate phase of education, many health care students are expected to conduct a project of one sort or another. They could (and we argued, should) involve insider practitioner research, with students critically appreciating aspects of practice they are experiencing. Qualified practitioners, we pointed out, are expected to undertake audit, and some engage in research. Since insider practitioner research would itself contribute to audit (and could even be claimed truly to be audit), time spent on this gains double value. Similarly, time spent in continuing professional development on attending conferences, and seminars, which rarely influence the development of practice (Davis *et al.*, 1995), could more usefully be spent on insider practitioner research. And the time currently spent (by some) on the preparation of clinical guidelines and protocols could similarly be used (we argued *more* profitably) (Davis *et al.*, 1995). Further, this work must be valued by key people within the organization, who also are professionals and whose expertise also lies beneath the surface. By conducting insider practitioner research *themselves*, they will come to recognize its value to them and to others. In this way, an 'evaluative culture' (Haines and Jones, 1994) will be created in which professionals are constantly looking at what they do and learning from this.

We believe there is an important role here for higher education. Traditionally this has been an academic function – to conduct research, to discover new knowledge, to promulgate the findings, and for practitioners to apply these to their practice. But this approach has failed to influence practice (Haines and Jones, 1994). As Stenhouse said in relation to the development of teaching in schools: academics have a contribution to make, 'but it is the teachers who in the end will change the world of the school by understanding it' (Stenhouse, 1975, p. 208). His vision was of schools 'as research and development institutions rather than clients of research and development agencies' (Stenhouse, 1975, p. 223). He saw the role of academics 'as helping schools to undertake research and development in a problem area and to report this work in a way that supports similar developments in other schools' (Stenhouse, 1975, p. 223). He added 'a research tradition which is accessible to teachers and which feeds teaching must be created if education is to be significantly improved' (Stenhouse,

1975, p. 165). We believe the same is true for the professions involved in health care. A similar tradition needs to be established. This will require a close partnership between academics and professional practitioners, a partnership of equals. But this requires a new approach by academics. Eraut talks of the need for higher education to be prepared 'to extend its role from that of creator and transmitter of generalizable knowledge to that of *enhancing the knowledge-creating capacities* of individuals and professional communities' (Eraut, 1994, p. 57).

Conclusion

Critical appreciation of practice, then, is both an individual enterprise and yet equally a profession-wide one, an individual and a collegiate one, a pre-registration (initial) and a post-registration (in-service education) matter. It involves the support of colleagues from higher education (to offer additional and wider perspectives) and one's immediate colleagues (to offer critical friendship), but also involves individual disciplined thinking and writing. It involves focusing on one's own practice and yet relating this particular to the wider field of the work of one's profession. It involves recognizing and fulfilling the demands of developing professional practice at the beginning of the course of professional preparation and continuing to attend to such matters until the end of one's career.

The benefits of critical appreciation lie for practitioners in the enriched understanding of their own practice and its professional traditions by means of learning to articulate its complexities. Such understanding will in turn gradually influence their practical work. As central to their professional development and in order to defend their professionalism, professionals need to be able to speak to fellow professionals and to lay persons (including clients and the guardians of the public interest) specifically about the details of the artistry of their practice, *in ways that are lacking in the literature cited in Chapter 3* and as a result contribute to the full appreciation of professional practice. This might also lead to the establishment on a broader base of a common language in which to discuss professional work, which would be particularly valuable in a multi-professional working situation which is rapidly becoming the norm in health care.

If professional practice truly develops when practitioners research their own practice, critical appreciation as a process in insider practitioner research should be at the heart of professional development. If this is so, then professional development based on critical appreciation needs a properly rigorous framework within which professionals can operate as appreciators of practice. How can such support be provided from within the research paradigms?

5

New directions in practitioner research: investigating *our* professional practice as *art*

Introduction

If as professionals we wish to investigate the *artistry* of our practice, a key question for us must be: by what approaches and methods – and thus within which research tradition – might we best do so? Given the important differences between art and science and the distinctive ways in which they operate, we are surely left querying the appropriateness of conducting enquiries into artistry from within a science or even a social science paradigm. Logic would seem to suggest that in neither the positivistic (scientific) nor in the interpretative and critical (social science) paradigms are the broad aims of research likely to be consonant with the aims of a practitioner exploring and investigating the artistry of his or her practice. To raise this issue does not imply a wish to replace one research paradigm with another, but merely to clarify the possibilities that each holds for the practitioner researcher. This is not about opposing science with art but about celebrating what art can offer differently from and in addition to science. This assumes that we are clear about the differences.

The nature of knowledge in art and science

Understanding the nature of the Arts by contrasting them to science, is not the same as suggesting that the Arts should replace science as the focus of our attention. Watson makes the point that it is crucial to know the functions that science cannot perform for understanding professional practice in health care and those that the humanities cannot perform in providing a knowledge base for a health care practitioner (Watson, 1985, p. 4). (Within the humanities here she subsumes the Arts.) She notes that 'science is concerned with methods, generalizations and predictions' while the humanities 'look for individual differences and uniqueness' and 'address themselves to understanding and the evaluation of human goals', and she adds that 'imagination and insight are validated from within, without justification by scientific criteria'. 'Science is not concerned with individual experience', but 'the humanities, on the other hand, cannot give predictable solutions to the problems of human nature. They cannot provide a hard data base of the intellectual propositional knowledge of a profession. Science and the Arts each have their own value system, and every individual practitioner has to relate to both of these while taking account of his or her own values' (Watson, 1985, p. 4).

Artistry, research and the nature of professional practice

As we have seen, the nature of professional practice is that much of it is (and always will be) ambiguous, messy, inexpressible and unmeasurable. The role of the artist (who works at understanding his or her own practice and the practice of art and artists more generally) is to enable us to notice the unrecognized, to see anew, to articulate the otherwise invisible and inexpressible. The character of the current research paradigms which offer the only accepted basis for recognized research is (as we shall see in more detail below) unalterably scientific – even where they challenge the world-view of the pure sciences and provide alternative 'interpretative' or 'critical' world-views. As a result, much work of the kind cited in Chapters 2 and 3 above is either unsupported as research (gaining no research grants, and even turned down as topics by university research committees) or is deemed something other than (and thus lower in status than) 'proper research'. Apart from preventing the construction and investigation of a balanced picture of practice, this view of artistry as having low status brings with it a more insidious danger, that when understandings about practice are cited by politicians and public, and when there are calls for practitioners to amass and harness the knowledge and understanding which research can offer to aid professional preparation and development, artistry will not be represented. Yet, it is inextricably part of professional practice.

The logic of this suggests that the artistry of practice should be investigated by means of research approaches drawn from the Arts. Since practitioners' investigations of their practice are essentially educational in nature (since they educate practitioners), and given the volume of work in this field as cited in Chapter 3, it seems reasonable to suggest that an artistic paradigm should be recognized within educational research which would provide a clearly worked out overall framework within which practitioner researchers could operate. Given that the recognition of an artistic research paradigm would allow for major developments in understanding professional practice and help to redress the balance of research work, this chapter attempts to show how such a paradigm might be delineated from current paradigms, and seeks to set these ideas within a practitioner research context.

The arguments here are about providing a framework within which professional practice can be investigated and understood in terms of the Arts, rather than about discussing professionals' work in terms of artistic theories (aesthetics). The concerns here are *centred* rather on the Arts than on hermeneutics or aesthetics. (Gadamer, for example, argues strongly for hermeneutics as a means of 'redressing the drawbacks of methodology's rule within the human sciences'; Watson and Chinn, 1994, p. 4.) He turns to poetry as offering access to greater truth and understanding than the human sciences, and his *Truth and Method* brings together classical studies, literary criticism, legal theory, philosophy and theology. His central investigation is into the nature of understanding in the humanities, rather than into practice in the Arts. He is interested in ideas and language, and particularly in aesthetics (see Gadamer, 1989). By contrast, given the principle of the primacy of practice and the possibilities for practitioners (as artists) to consider their practice in the terms in which artists consider theirs, it is the recognition of an artistic (not an aesthetic) paradigm in educational research that is being argued for here. The terminology is important. It does not exclude aesthetics, but indicates that the major investigative focus is the *practical achievements of artistry*, in professional work, not (although they are related) *ideas about art and the meaning of art and life*. Indeed, given the work cited in Chapter 3 above, it is possible to argue that an arts paradigm of this very kind has long since existed in practitioner research in all but name.

What is being explored in this chapter, then, is not the recognition of a new paradigm designed to replace others, but one which is operated alongside others, which will enrich our ability to understand practice and provide more appropriately for capturing and exploring the complexity of practice. The word 'paradigm' ('world-view') indicates a self-standing system of ideas which reinforce each other and constitute a whole and independent system of thought. Research is conducted by working within or drawing upon such a system of ideas, which enables researchers to show that their work is properly rigorous. However, it is also recognized that any one paradigm will not alone be sufficient to enable us to do justice to the complexity of professional practice. Rather, these ways of thinking about the world of practice need to be drawn upon rigorously and appropriately by a professional wishing to understand practice and who arguably should seek, *while using eclectically their methods and means*, to *honour the world-view* (paradigm) from which they are drawn. Thus, for example, the practitioner researcher, working on a small scale, is likely to draw upon a range of paradigms, but set the investigation within a case study or action research framework. If such an *approach* could be informed by and draw upon an artistic paradigm as well as those paradigms which have hitherto provided methods for such studies, this would redress a current imbalance. The details of how this might operate in practice are the subject of Part Three.

In order to explore the likely details of an artistic research paradigm, this chapter is divided into three main sections. The first attempts to clarify the meaning of practitioner research, since the new paradigm being outlined is essentially of use to those in professional practice. The second section offers, as an *aide-mémoire*, a review summary of the current traditional educational research paradigms (the positivist paradigm and its alternatives, the interpretative and the critical) and seeks to indicate their contributions to the work of practitioners. In relation to these, the third section explores in the same detail the character of a putative artistic paradigm of educational research. This chapter thus prepares the way for Part Three, which looks in detail at using an artistic paradigm in practice.

Practitioner research

What is practitioner research? Who are practitioner researchers? They are professionals who are 'part of the world that they are researching' and who 'have a history and a future in that culture' which they are investigating (Reed and Procter, 1995, p. 5). They are professionals who recognize the need of practitioners to understand their *own* practice and the practical problems of their work, and to consider them critically within the history and traditions of the practical work of their profession. The subject of practitioner research is thus professional practice itself, and the intention is to extend the understanding of it. Such understanding provides the basis and the potential to change practitioners' ways of seeing their work and thereby to develop individual professional practice and ultimately to develop the work of the profession as a whole.

Practitioner research and practitioner knowledge

It should be noted that this notion takes for granted the idea that practising professionals have a peculiar and important form of knowledge (professional knowledge) which is intrinsically different from – but is not inferior to – knowledge created by scientific research, and which shapes decisions about *what* to research (which identifies what needs to be better understood) and considers *how* it should be researched. Reed and Procter (1995, p. 23) argue that to improve practice and professional knowledge is to 'articulate the voice of the experienced practitioner and explicate the tacit knowledge that is embedded in practice'. Although they do not say so, the most difficult aspect of tacit knowledge to explore is the artistry of practice. They suggest the broad Aristotelian distinctions also discussed in Fish and Coles (1998) – that the major difference between practitioner research and 'traditional' (scientific) research is that the end result of practitioner research is practical (procedural) and relates to understanding about practice, whereas the end result of the scientific research is essentially theoretical and relates to propositional (factual) knowledge, which practitioners are left to apply in order to turn it into something practical. This latter kind of research is, therefore, not strictly practitioner research, though it still may be research *for* practitioners. As a result, practitioner research is more often likely to be based within or to draw heavily upon the alternative rather than the scientific paradigms. Indeed, it is even doubtful whether scientific research can ever shape in a major way the work of practitioner researchers.

Practitioner research and reflective practice

The practitioner researcher, then, is the practitioner who investigates his or her own practice in properly rigorous ways which are open to public scrutiny. And intrinsic in this is that we are rarely able to give an accurate commentary upon our activities, but almost inevitably employ as part of our capturing of practice *ex post facto* reasoning and rationalizing. As we have seen already, however, this does not prevent the development of new understandings arising both during the process and from the final narrative and its subsequent interrogation. The practitioner researcher is to be contrasted with the researcher who enquires into that practice from *outside* it and can thus never be privy to most of what we characterized as the nine-tenths of the iceberg of our practice which is below the visible surface (see, p. 99). The practitioner researcher is also to be contrasted with that particular kind of so-called reflective practitioner who eschews the notion of *investigating* practice rigorously and who merely adopts a ritualistic and superficial way of 'thinking back' over (reconstructing) recent activities, and who having done so, closes the subject. A practitioner researcher who systematically takes an investigative stance towards practice has the best chance of uncovering the highly subjective elements of his or her professional work, and by recognizing them as such makes them the subject of further study and personal professional development.

Outsider and insider researchers

Reed and Procter usefully offer a continuum of what they call researcher positions, from 'outsider researcher' (one who undertakes research into practice with no professional experience), through a 'hybrid researcher' (an unfortunately scientific metaphor for one who undertakes research into the practice of other practitioners) to 'insider researcher' ('a practitioner who undertakes research into their own and their colleagues' practice') (Reed and Procter, 1995, p. 10). Clearly, a practitioner researcher will normally be what is here called an 'insider researcher', though he or she might also work in the hybrid category.

However, the notion of the insider practitioner researcher brings with it the notion that a practitioner's subjective and 'insider's' view is likely to be somehow blurred by subjectivity, whereas the outside researcher's view is clear, objective, accurate and clean, and that 'proper research' must be large scale in nature (a view promoted by the Research Assessment Exercises which have bedevilled our universities in the 1990s). But such insider practitioner research, values 'noise' in the scientific system which contributes to self-understanding (Kemmis, 1995, pp. 3–4). Practitioner research operating in the alternative paradigms is, therefore, not a weak form of research, but merely a different form, strong in some aspects where other forms of research are weak and which makes a significant contribution to understanding professional practice. Indeed, practitioner research has been shown to have a much greater impact upon practitioners than other forms of research (see Beeston and Simons, 1996; Fish and Coles, 1998).

There are, however, some misconceptions embedded in the popular notion of individual, insider practitioner research. These include the idea that 'reflection' is the same as thinking about one's practice, that people 'do it all the time', and that good practitioners have always done it. For some this leads to the equally unsupportable belief that any kind of description of a piece of practice containing a few concluding points about how (in the light of this) *others* ought to operate, is both reflection and research. Thus arises the assumption that reflection can be equated with a (lower) form of research in its own right. In fact it is not research at all if it is not demonstrably systematic and rigorous and its methods are not publicly open to critical scrutiny. What then, counts, and what should count, as research?

Research and its paradigms

The kind of research that practitioners most frequently conduct in order to enlighten their practice, since it is designed to educate them, is located within the research traditions of *educational* research. This is traditionally seen as falling broadly into quantitative and qualitative research, and then into specific paradigms.

Depending on how professional practice is seen, so it is researched, investigated, and practised. This has given rise to three key research paradigms (whole and independent systems of ideas) or traditions, in which researcher and practitioner see themselves as working: the positivist, the interpretative and the critical. Although of course, as Hoyle and John point out, 'much of the research and thinking done in relation to . . . professional knowledge rarely draws on one tradition exclusively' (Hoyle and John, 1995, p. 56).

In seeking an appropriate approach to investigating a chosen topic, there are many decisions researchers have to make and argue for in relation to their intentions for that subject, themselves and their audience, in order to work with rigour. These include: which research paradigm to operate within, or to utilize, or draw upon for specific sections of the research; which approaches within that to adopt; which methodology and what tools to utilize (how to capture, process and present the data or evidence); and what kinds of conclusion it is therefore appropriate to come to. Such decisions should be guided by overall research intentions, by resources available and by the view of professional practice held by the researcher, as well as the deeper issues associated with this decision-making process (for example about the validity and reliability of the work, and the nature of evidence).

It should be noted that some of the content in each of the three following sections, particularly the paragraph in each section which summarizes details about the paradigm and the tables which follow, have been influenced by the work of W. Carr, 1995, pp. 90–99. I also acknowledge helpful discussion of an early draft of Table 5.1 with Colin Coles.

Quantitative research

Quantitative research is concerned with empirical matters. In its classical scientific form its procedures are based upon the pure sciences, starting from *theory* – a hypothesis – which must be test-able and replicable, providing an explanation which is generaliz-able. However, there is also a 'macro-sociological' version which concerns itself with very large scale surveys which look at practices in relation to historical, economic and cultural contexts, recording observable facts and behaviours on a grand scale and in relation to grand theories (for example, Marxism) in order to make sense of the data. Quantitative research is normally conducted by profes-sional researchers (not professional practitioners) and it is con-cerned strictly with systematic recording of empirical matters from an objective angle. As its name suggests, it focuses on collecting data related to the measurement of the visible with a view to ana-lysing this, generalizing from it and thus creating new knowledge which can be prescribed for application by educators and practi-tioners. This is not to suggest that some figures and empirical mat-ters are of no interest at all in qualitative research, but that the intentions and focus of qualitative research are different.

The scientific or positivist research paradigm
To those for whom the foundation of their professional practice is predominantly their propositional (factual) knowledge, research and development is seen as having the duty to extend that kind of knowledge. For them the scientific or positivist paradigm is of cen-tral importance and use, and they rely upon it to produce more and more up-to-date information which they can acquire and then put into practice. It has certainly left its mark on health care profes-sionals, many of whom have been brought up to believe that it is the only kind of research. Indeed, it is deeply embedded in our subconscious as 'the only proper research' (and this view has been further entrenched by the universities' Research Assessment Exer-cise which constructs league tables of how much *scientific* research lecturers have done and then hands out funds to universities accordingly).

The positivist research paradigm has represented for several cen-turies the prevailing view of the way to conduct research. It seeks truth and is useful for those who want to know facts about their world and who see the world of practice as yielding to scientific study. Its methods are those of the pure sciences. It seeks to dis-cover unassailable empirical evidence in order to prove theories by means of fact and logic. Its focus is thus on a rigorous collecting and then analysing and classifying of large scale empirical data, in order to generalize from it. It is, thus, reductionist. Its intentions are for researchers to produce hitherto unknown or unrecognized factual knowledge for practitioners to apply to their practical work. Its virtues are its objectivity and its ability to handle large amounts of evidence, and from these to uncover new knowledge.

In scientific research, then, the task is to discover value-free (that is, objective), law-like (and context-free) generalizations. These might offer a new basis for practice which practitioners themselves have actually not sought or (sometimes) it might provide 'answers' to practitioners' problems and enable the activities of professional practice to become more efficient. (The problem here, as we have seen in Chapters 1 and 2, is that there are always unique elements in practitioners' work which do not yield to large scale generalization.) The belief, however, is that possession of such research knowledge will at last allow practitioners to take their rightful place as professionals.

It should be noted too that this view brings with it acceptance of (what many see as) a highly unfortunate divide between researchers and practitioners. It could in fact be argued that this view of professional practice has proved and is still proving unhelpful in promoting significant professional development precisely because of this divide, since it puts theory and research before practice, it eschews attitudes and values in a fruitless attempt to be objective and it places over-riding emphasis on the impossible task of producing context-free laws (which are rarely useful in highly idiosyncratic situations).

In outline then the scientific paradigm is derived from the natural sciences (particularly, as Hamilton *et al.* (1977, p. 7) pointed out, the agricultural–botanical sciences). The main purpose of such research is to produce propositional knowledge. The researchers are research professionals, who must be objective, neutral and in no way associated with the arena they are researching, being outsiders to the profession as well as to the setting of the research. The audience consists of fellow academic researchers, practitioners who are expected to apply this new knowledge to practice, and politicians who gain from it (often simplistic and frequently revised) answers to simplistic questions or legitimation for the requirements they make of practitioners in respect of what they should do and what they should know. The view of theory and practice is that theory is pre-eminent, that it should come first (as a hypothesis) and should structure what is sought in the practical arena. The data from practice (after being processed – which is also guided by theory) are then used to form further theories. The underlying metaphor is of 'moulding' practice by theory. Methods, drawn from the natural sciences, are experimental, quantitative and analytic. This includes large scale experiments using control groups (randomized controlled trials) and formal evaluation studies utilizing notional standards, based on a system of pre-tests, new processes and post-tests. The data sought are those which will provide evidence for proving the hypothesis with which the research begins. They involve clear-cut, simple, large scale information and the intention is to turn this into generalized facts and figures. Measurement is all. The view of knowledge is that it can be reduced to clear and objective information, and that evidence must consist of that which is visible, the truth of which must be unassailable (differing interpretations are not tolerated). The proof to which this all leads must be (so far as can be known) absolute. Rigour is achieved via a research design which ensures that the work is valid (that the enquiry does indeed provide the data and evidence that it purports to and is not contaminated by elements that distort its intentions and processes), and by ensuring its reliability (such that later researchers could replicate it). In such research the values inherent in decisions and behaviours of researchers and researched are excluded from consideration, and moral issues do not impinge centrally on the research activities, but are set to one side for consideration by others (often practitioners) (see Table 5.1).

Qualitative research

Qualitative research, by contrast to, and as a radical alternative to, the quantitative approach, was developed originally within the social sciences, and starts with *practice*, and works towards uncovering theory. Here, currently, are two major paradigms. The first is the interpretative paradigm, where ethnomethodological methods of anthropology (participant observation and interviewing) are used and which looks at opinions and perceptions and at the perspectives and relationships of participants – usually through case study.

Qualitative research: the interpretative paradigm

By contrast to the view that the world of professional practice (like all other aspects of the world) could best be explored through the positivistic paradigm, there exists the alternative notion that professional work in all arenas is a social practice (Golby, 1993; Langford, 1985), and that it is properly explored through social science. Here both the term 'social' and the term 'practice' are significant, and the research processes used by practitioners and the ends to which they can be put are of interest to researcher and practitioner alike. Indeed, in this view the professional practitioner and the researcher may be one and the same person. This paradigm seeks understanding of issues and processes related to both theory and practice. Here a range of perspectives is sought, and a range of interpretations is expected. Here the concern is not so much with creating new knowledge but with understanding a particular practice within its wider professional practice context, with acknowledging professional responsibilities to clients, with recognizing the values base of professional work and the moral dimensions of it, with improving professional practice by recognizing the traditions within which it operates and with the importance of enabling practitioners to theorize their practice. This paradigm seeks to enlighten practice and aid decision-making about its complex moral basis (see Eraut, 1994, who discusses these matters in detail).

In order to be compared with the scientific paradigm, the following outline of the interpretative paradigm is offered. The derivation of such research is in the disciplines of the social sciences (particularly anthropology, especially its branches of phenomenology and ethnomethodology). The main focus of such research, then, is the description and interpretation of specific social settings, and its form is subjective. The practical purpose is to inform and deepen, illuminate and enhance understanding of the social setting (in the complex world of professional practice), by means of discovering and documenting aspects of the social world it is studying, and recognizing recurring patterns and flushing out individual differences and critical perspectives. The researchers here are either research professionals or practising professionals, who gain or who have extensive access to the practical setting. The audience consists of practitioners who themselves are seeking the good of their professional clients and whose understanding will be enhanced by the research but who will never be expected directly to 'apply' what has been found in one setting to another. (They are practitioners who have some control over their professional lives.) The primacy of practice is a key principle.

Such research begins by looking at the practical setting with a relatively open mind. Theory emerges from practice, and relevant formal theory is brought up to that practice. The underlying metaphor is of 'growth' of understanding about practice. Methods are drawn from the social sciences and are qualitative and interpretative. Examples include: observation (structured and unstructured, participant and non-participant); the capturing of interaction (structured and unstructured); interviews (semi-structured and in-depth); field notes; diaries; documentary analysis; situational analysis. This paradigm finds its expression in descriptive or deliberative case study and/or in some (properly systematic) forms of reflective practice. The data sought are acknowledged as complex and human, and are recognized as not yielding to simplistic processing. The view of knowledge is that it is complex, muddied at all points by motives, values and moral dilemmas and is thus no more than tentative and far from being able to be reduced to clear and objective information. This view of research conceives of evidence as at best evidence of only one small example, which is a particular version of practice and which can only be related to more general issues as a specific example of a general case. There is no proof, knowledge being tentative. The research however is endorsed by the reverberation of recognition in the reader. Rigour is achieved via multiple perspectives, the idea being that at least three distinct sighting points are needed in order to see something three dimensional in all its facets. It is also achieved by means of frequent checking of the researchers' perceptions with those of the research subjects. In such research the values inherent in decisions and behaviours of researchers and researched are central to consideration, and moral issues impinge centrally on the research activities (see Table 5.1).

This, then, is the interpretative view. It is about understanding, describing and being able to explain the social world and those who inhabit it 'in terms of their . . . inner realms of human consciousness' (Hoyle and John, 1995, p. 55). Here motivation and intention are as significant as observable behaviour, and the moral responsibilities of the professional are ever present. Here values and attitudes are at the heart of the research and are recognized and highlighted as the research progresses. The end here is the improvement of understanding of professional practice and the consequent change the practitioner researcher is trusted to effect is the well-founded improvement of practice – but in due time, not as a knee-jerk reaction. It is thus antithetical to our present climate of short-termism and has rated as of low status in the universities' Research Assessment Exercise in many (though not all) universities. Its value for some practitioners is however very considerable, allowing them to channel their energy into achieving the possible. But for others it is essentially conservative, accepting what it cannot change and working on only what it can easily affect.

Qualitative research: the critical paradigm

By contrast to the interpretative paradigm, the critical paradigm starts with an intention of emancipating practitioners from the power relationships in which they are involved by engaging them in 'praxis' where both the theory and practice which operate in the practical setting come under investigation and critical scrutiny and a critique of practice is constructed, so that the enlightenment it offers transforms the consciousness of the practitioner. Thus, it specifically promotes critical thinking and reflection. This version of qualitative research is conducted mainly by practitioners (usually looking at their own practice) and takes an admittedly subjective stance to its subjects. Being founded on the social sciences, it seeks to capture the quality of and the complexity of life in small scale social settings, to interpret these in a range of ways, and to produce new ways of understanding, and thus *developing* the work of practitioners.

For those who see professional practice as a political activity, in terms of its social, economic and political bases or who are concerned with feminism, who wish to achieve greater change than is promised by either of the previous two paradigms and who seek to focus centrally on the values implicit in their views, there is a dissatisfaction with the positivist and the interpretative traditions. For them the critical paradigm offers more highly interventionist ways of thinking and acting in relation to professional practice. It even offers a notion that professional practice and research (the practitioner researcher him or herself) can change more than simply the practitioner's immediate world. It is based upon critical social science and finds its main practitioner expression in action research or critical case study. Here, all forms of (empirical) investigation of social contexts are harnessed eclectically. And the audience is the practitioners themselves as well as their organization and its managers, and – ultimately – politicians.

The following outline of the critical paradigm is offered to facilitate comparison with the scientific and interpretative ones. The derivation of such research is in the disciplines of the social and political sciences. The main focus of such research is critical and transformative, and the practical purpose is to provide a more critical base for the development of professional knowledge and thus to emancipate the professional. The researchers involved are most likely to be insider practitioner researchers who may use critical case study research or action research as their main approach. The research is primarily aimed at practitioners, their organization and management and politicians at a range of levels. The primacy of practice is a key principle, but the work is in fact strongly shaped by Aristotelian philosophy in respect of praxis and by Critical Theory (an aspect of Marxist ideology and not to be confused with literary theory or with critical appreciation of the Arts). The underlying metaphor is emancipation from the uncritical acceptance of theory and practice. Methods are broadly the same as for the interpretative paradigm but in this case are designed to investigate the problematic in both theory and practice and to contribute to the development of a fundamental critique of both by encouraging new meaning-making in the practical arena. The data sought are those that will contribute to the dialectical debate about problematic issues. Here knowledge is defined as being socially, economically and politically constructed and 'therefore tied to fundamental structural interests' (Hoyle and John, 1995, p. 55), and evidence of this is sought but truth is recognized as complex and proof is not a concern. Rather, the force of dialectical argument is of major significance. Rigour is achieved via multiple perspectives. Here the values inherent in decisions and behaviours of both researchers and researched, as well as the moral issues, are seen from within a political framework (see Table 5.1).

It is interesting to observe that where professional practice is increasingly prescribed by bureaucrats from outside the profession, this emancipatory view of research tends to gain more support from working practitioners who see their professionalism threatened. But it is not necessarily the guardian of the only good, and like any other form of research, it does not always deliver what it promises – in this case because individuals cannot always transform given forms of social life.

The possibility of an artistic research paradigm

None of the paradigms described above, however, takes account of all that we have said in the previous chapters about professional practice as an artistic activity. We saw it as characterized by the wish not to separate theory and practice; not to atomize the elements of the practice setting; not to overlook but to recognize and find language for the elements of practice which are mysterious, ineffable; not to ignore or fear uncertainty and error, but to use them creatively. We saw this as much more akin to the processes of the Arts. How, then, might practitioner research be enabled to take professional artistry much more seriously? What can be learnt from the Arts? The following is an attempt to respond to this. It does so by drawing upon investigations conducted into professional artistry as outlined in Chapter 3 and as found in Chinn and Watson (1994), Eisner (1993, 1995), Fish and Coles (1998) and Schön (1987a). None of this work, however, had the support of a fully worked out artistic research paradigm.

Where traditional research operates within the scientific/ empirical paradigm, and social science research takes place in either the interpretative/empirical or the critical/political paradigms, this new proposal is for an artistic/holistic paradigm. This signals that it draws upon the disciplines of the Arts to enlighten the artistry of practice (to recognize, express and investigate the otherwise inexpressible qualities of professional practice) and that it is concerned with the appreciation of practice and particularly that it is interested in responding holistically to the artistry under scrutiny. Here we begin to see that we are entering a quite different world from the empirical world of the sciences and social sciences. Here there are quite different ways of thinking about professional practice, and there are different questions to be asked and methods available to be used. For example, the values inherent in the decisions and behaviours of researchers and researched are central to the holistic view of practice in this paradigm. *Value* is itself at the core of such appreciation. (See Part Three for more detail on how this operates in practice.) And there is an interest in moral issues here. Our moral concerns come into play when we read about or see moral insights depicted in drama, literature or painting. Indeed, the Arts offer a key means of exploring moral matters.

The derivation of the artistic/holistic paradigm is to be found in the disciplines of literature, drama, music and art. The main focus of the artistic/holistic paradigm is recognizing and responding to, understanding *and valuing*, the artistry of professional practice. Its human interest is in the appreciation and connoisseurship of good practice, with a view to making it generally possible to enable people to 'make such appreciation their own' (to experience that appreciation from the inside, rather than being dependent on the judgement of others). Its practical purpose is to inform professional judgement as it is operated within professional practice; to enable professional judgements to be made about professional practice as displayed and discussed within validation, accreditation, evaluation exercises and even inspectorial activities, as well as staff development arenas; and to celebrate good practice and thus to inspire (different) artistry in others. (It is not for copying.) The researcher would need to be a practitioner and an insider, and the audience is practitioners and their clients, course validators and accreditors, evaluators, inspectors and the public who are increasingly wishing to discuss and influence professional practice. The view in this paradigm of theory and practice is that they are inseparable. The focus of this kind of research is the practice setting.

Perhaps one of the greatest differences from other sorts of research that working in this paradigm brings, is the overall nature of the way it is conducted. Both the scientific and the social sciences paradigms require a meticulously pre-planned research design which states clearly and in detail beforehand what will be achieved, and which places much emphasis on the pre-planning of every method and procedure to be utilized in that achievement. By comparison, the artistic paradigm recognizes that uncovering the complexity of human situations which themselves cannot be entirely pre-planned (involving as they do activities like improvisation, or making on-the-spot judgements) can only be achieved by keeping open for as long as possible the processes to be used and the questions to be asked.

The main processes of research in the artistic/holistic paradigm would include the constructing of a literary portrait of practice (following the making of a number of draft pictures of practice) together with the production of a critical commentary on that portrait and (via the portrait), on the original practice. The portrait or narrative of practice would attempt to be faithful to overall impression and visible facts as well as to nuance and the elements of artistry involved. It would also be sensitive to theories-in-use as they occur in the piece of practice focused upon (and is likely to employ means drawn not only from the practitioners' espoused theories and from a range of formal theories but also particularly from the Arts, to enable the more ineffable elements of that practice to be articulated). The critical commentary would be developed by as many means as possible and would be focused first on the portrait and, via it, the original piece of practice. The only data here are the various drafts of the portrait of practice that are produced on the way to the final version, together with any information collected before, during or after the construction of the narrative of practice to enrich (rather than sanitize) that portrait and further enlighten the commentary on it (via interview, documentary analysis or situational analysis). This is most likely to include various attempts to check with those involved in the practice setting how they too viewed it.

The underlying view of human nature in such a paradigm is that practitioners are responsive to the creative impetus within themselves (which can be stimulated by consideration of critical thinking about art) and are also able to gain understanding and ultimately seek to achieve better practice themselves through experiencing and responding to the creative artefacts of others. The underlying metaphors are of liberation – ultimately from the vision of others – via imagination (imagination being a key ability which characterizes artistic practice), and of strength – in formulating and refining one's own vision – via learning to value good practice (because individuals who gain understanding of their own and of others' practice are in a position to develop and refine their work for themselves). In this way the artistic/holistic paradigm is highly moralistic (since it drives towards learning to value a good and as a result to act to produce a good.) As Armstrong says of appreciating painting:

> appreciation spins out into behaviour and life. If I am ready to appreciate the value of something, I must be prepared to value it

above other things. I must say that it is more important than something else, and I must act in line with this. This is an aspect of really
finding something valuable, and not just asserting that one does.
(Armstrong, 1996, p. 26)

In this sense, the artistic/holistic paradigm would offer an interesting way forward for the new intentions for professional development proposed by D. Carr (1995) and Hagar (1997). They argue
for professional development to focus on the processes of acquiring
the capacity to exercise Aristotelian (practical) widsom. Following
Aristotle, they see these as: developing the habit of acting justly
through following the advice of elders, thus learning the attraction
and pleasure of acting virtuously; learning therefore which actions
are virtuous, but not understanding why; and ultimately attaining
practical wisdom in full by practising and exploring the nature
of that practice. In each of these stages, 'cognitive, practical and
emotional elements are significantly intertwined' (Hagar, 1997, p.
115). Such intertwining might best be appreciated through the
approach offered in the artistic/holistic paradigm.

Methods for the artistic/holistic paradigm are drawn from the
creative processes in the Arts – particularly story-telling and painting, together with the recognized discipline of appreciation of these
arts (what are sometimes called critical appreciation, or practical
criticism, or critical commentary of performance and of text).
These involve a knowledge of form and structure, language and
style, tone and mood, meaning and symbol, as considered in Part
Two. The *detail* of how these are able to be utilized to research
professional practice is considered in Part Three. The view of
knowledge is that practitioner knowledge – as captured in the iceberg metaphor – is most significant. Of the nine-tenths that is invisible to an observer, some is entirely unable to be reduced to clear
and objective information based upon factual evidence, but it is
able to be recognized and responded to. It is this large proportion
of practice that the artistic/holistic paradigm is *particularly* interested in. But the artistic/holistic researcher's interest is in the context
of the appreciation of the practice as a whole concept and not as
something that can be isolated and atomized. This work depends
not upon proof, but persuasion and upon the recognition by others
of the 'artistic truth' that is being presented (just as a reader
responds to a novel or poem by recognizing in it something which

they knew at a deep level). (This is referred to as 'inter-subjective validity', see Chapter 11, p. 253.) It is not scientific truth that is being sought in this paradigm but artistic truth, which sometimes reaches far deeper issues. Rigour here is achieved in the discipline of the writing, that it is as close as possible to capturing the 'whole iceberg' of a piece of practice and particularly the artistry involved in that practice. In such research the values inherent in decisions and behaviours of researchers and researched are central, and moral issues are as described above. (See Table 5.1 for the contrast of this paradigm to those previously discussed.)

Distinguishing artistic/holistic practitioner research from work in the Arts

It is however a fair question (particularly where an artistic research paradigm is being argued for) to seek the differences between practitioner research and, say, journalism, novels or short stories. In terms of the artefact produced (the story or picture), the line between the two can appear at first sight very thin. Besides which, for both the professional practitioner and the artist, the activities are highly personal and the background interest is in developing their own practice. See, for example, Golby (1993) on case study (where journalistic case studies are cited as examples), and Groundwater-Smith (1984) where the differences between faction and fiction are discussed. But the researcher, in the rigour with which he or she seeks to capture specific practice and in the critical perspectives offered in the commentary, will produce more than just an artistic end product.

It is also possible to distinguish clearly between the overall intention of the artist and that of the practitioner. The researcher is intent upon laying hold of an understanding of his or her practice. This goes beyond portraying and capturing and requires recourse to critique also – which artists can leave to their audience. Further, there are different starting points – different origins, with differing impetuses and with different emotions. The artist starts with some chosen or accepted inspiration (which may be imagined or real), some vision of a part of the world – some view of it – which he or she recognizes and feels impelled to capture and usually to offer to others so that they too may see it that way. The practitioner starts

Table 5.1 Four research paradigms

Characteristics	Scientific/positivistic	Humanistic/interp'tive	Critical/political	Artistic/holistic
Derivation	The natural sciences (botany)	The social sciences (anthropology)	The social and political sciences	The Arts (music, art, literature)
Main focus	The technical and scientific	Description and interpretation	Critique and transformation	Understanding and valuing good practice
Practical purpose	To produce new propositional knowledge	To inform and deepen understanding of social settings	To provide a more political base for professional change	To inform practitioners' judgements and appreciation of practice
Origin of researcher	The world of professional research	Professional researchers and practitioners	Most likely to be insider practitioner researchers	Insider practitioner researchers
Audience	Other researchers, practitioners (to apply new ideas), public and politicians	Professional practitioners and researchers	Practitioners and their organization and management, also politicians	Practitioners, and all who judge them
View of theory and practice	Theory is pre-eminent	The primacy of practice is a key principle	Primacy of practice, ideas of praxis, Marxist ideology	Primacy of practice as a holistic idea
Underlying metaphor	Moulding	Growth	Emancipation	Enlightenment and liberation via imagination
Approach	Randomized controlled trials	Descriptive case study	Deliberative and critical case study	Appreciation

Methods	Experimental quantitative analytic Large scale	Observation, interaction, interview, field notes, diaries Small scale	Observation, interaction, interview, field notes, diaries Small scale	Creative arts processes Narrative and critical commentary Small scale
Data sought	Clear-cut, large scale, suitable for turning into figures Measurement is all	Complex human data Data does not yield to simple reduction	Designed to investigate the problematic in both theory and practice	Only that which enlightens narrative and supports commentary
View of knowledge and evidence	Knowledge is always reducible to clear and objective information Evidence is empirical and unproblematic	Complex, muddied by values and moral dilemmas, and so at best tentative Small scale evidence is unable to be generalized	Practical knowledge is made in situ Evidence is value-based	Practitioner knowledge needs developing Evidence is via recognition by others
View of truth and proof	Truth is unassailable Proof can be watertight	Problematic, but endorsed by the recognition of practitioners	Problematic and political, endorsed by practitioners' recognition	Artistic truth is deeper than scientific truth, and suits the iceberg of practice
Means of achieving rigour	Designing research to ensure validity and reliability	Use of multiple perspectives	Use of multiple perspectives	The rigour is in the discipline of the writing and is judged in terms of artistic values
Values inherent in the research	Values excluded from design Moral considerations are for others, not for researchers	Values central Moral considerations impinge at all points	Values central Moral considerations central	Values central Moral issues and aesthetic values

with a given piece of practice – with what has really happened – and probably with something that called attention to itself because of some unease. And he or she then works towards a holistic vision of it. In addition, there are different processes involved. The researcher, as a professional practitioner working within the traditions of his or her profession, strives to be both an artist and a critic – a producer of narratives and portraits but also an interrogator of them, in coming to a greater understanding of his or her own practice. The artist, by contrast, works from within an artistic tradition to produce an artefact that aptly conveys his or her vision. Further, the artist's work may be shrouded in secrecy during the process of creation, but then is revealed to the public, and the artist then usually leaves to the wide and unknown audience the appreciation of his or her creation. By contrast, the practitioner works in ways that will be considered and weighed by a critical professional audience *and* the public. And in respect of the end result, the practitioner becomes (along with immediate fellow professionals) essentially his or her own audience.

The foregoing has offered ideas which have perforce been about the principles of research. Rather more detail of ways of working within this new paradigm is offered in Part Three. First, however, it is necessary to examine in more detail the language and processes involved in recognizing and responding to art and artistry, in order to use them as a starting point for the practical ideas which then follow.

Part Two

Recognition and response: the traditions and practices of critical appreciation in the Arts

6

The language of appreciation 1: seeing and reading

Introduction to Part Two

This part of the book focuses on ideas endemic to, and language used in, the critical appreciation of the Arts. Its intention is to offer support – or one starting point – for those attempting to capture and discuss the artistry of professional practice and produce a critical appreciation of it (or to read those of others). It seeks to help them to develop or extend their understanding of some processes of creation in the Arts and to establish a wide repertoire of language and ideas about the Arts. This is not so that they can *apply* these to practice, but so that they can draw on them to illuminate practice.

It was argued in Part One that seeing professional practice *as artistry* is a means of recognizing its entire character (by comparison with the narrow technical rational view that is interested only in skills and those elements of practice which are readily visible). At the end of Chapter 2 were listed a number of characteristics commonly found in professional practice which would be excluded if a narrow technical rational view were to be adopted. Taking a holistic view of professional practice, then, the practitioner can be seen as an artist. These notions were reinforced in Chapter 3 where a range of literature from across the caring professions provided much evidence that, despite the inimical climate, professional practice is increasingly recognized in terms of artistry, and the practitioner is seen as a maker of meanings (in the practice setting and afterwards) through language which comes essentially from the

Arts and critical appreciation in the Arts. Further, arguments were offered in Chapter 4 for career-long professional development which seeks a holistic understanding of professional activities and which relies for much of this on the ability to produce a critical appreciation of practice (which is also useful for fulfilling the demands of accountability and quality assurance). As we shall see in detail in Part Three, such an appreciation might include both a portrait of an example of practice and a critical commentary on that portrait and (through it) on the practice itself.

Accordingly, Part Two focuses on specific examples of the Arts and offers perspectives on the language and ideas endemic to appreciating them critically. Chapter 6 discusses particular examples of literature and painting, where the audience is involved in seeing or reading, and the creator is involved in using words and pictures. These activities are also those of professional practitioners. Such activities have considerable relevance to professionals' work, to their capturing of it in a portrait (in words) and their producing a commentary on it and on the work of their profession more generally. Such a commentary or critique, as we have seen earlier, goes beyond what is required of an artist. Chapter 7 focuses on the performance arts in order to consider the language appropriate to a critical appreciation of performance – since much of practitioners' work involves performance – and in order to discuss some matters associated with this.

Subscribing to an unashamedly old-fashioned stance, the term 'art' in these two chapters is taken to mean that which has been generally accorded recognition as having intrinsic merit and which in that way is considered as beyond the ordinary, in visual art, music, film, dance, literature (poetry, prose – including biography and autobiography as well as novel, novella and short story – and drama). 'Having intrinsic merit' is taken to mean having a significant and recognizable, individual and unique character which is the result of the maker's personal vision (which vision is offered from within a particular tradition but which, as we shall see, is susceptible to individual interpretation). Further, the accolade 'art' is taken to indicate that the maker of an artefact so described has drawn upon imagination, and produced an invention which can be recognized as combining style and content in a unity, so that the whole makes new meanings, forges new connections and enables us to see the world anew. Such an artistic invention (as Horace said) both delights and teaches, and its teaching has a moral dimension, where the invented world has much to say about the real world and the 'maker' conveys more than has been said explicitly.

Introduction to Chapter 6

The chapter is divided into two main sections. It begins with specific examples of work in the Arts rather than with theories about the Arts. Here some concrete examples of the Arts are presented (these are: a story, together with a brief digression to a novel, a painting and a poem) and a critical appreciation of each is offered. By reference to these examples, the second section reviews the language of appreciation, presenting firstly a number of concepts common to all the Arts, and then exploring the language of literature and of painting. Professional practitioners should bear in mind while reading this chapter that the processes of capturing and thinking critically about their work will involve telling the story of their practice as well as standing back from it and responding to it. The following is therefore of central significance for them.

Exploring some specific examples of the Arts

In order to offer concrete examples of literature and painting for the sake of exploring issues related to observing, writing and reading, I have chosen three which are inter-related in overall subject matter (overt surface topics) and which share common themes (underlying issues) but which offer us three very different art forms. Both subject and themes seem particularly relevant. The underlying themes are suffering and the development of the artist and artistry. The subject matter for all three is based upon the story of Daedalus and Icarus. Daedalus was a craftsman of unique talent who constructed the Cretan Labyrinth for King Minos. His name today is synonymous with artifice (the dictionary offers Daedalian as 'displaying artistic skill, formed with art, intricate and varied'). The pieces of art chosen are: the story of Daedalus and Icarus (with a brief nod at the fact that the hero of James Joyce's *Portrait of the Artist as a Young Man* (Joyce, 1967 [1916]) is very deliberately called Stephen Daedalus); Bruegel the Elder's painting *Landscape with the Fall of Icarus*; and W. H. Auden's poem 'Musée des Beaux Arts'.

In offering these examples to the reader, I shall do little more than *present what is there* in each of these three differing particular pieces of art. My aim is to do no more than aid the reader in looking very carefully at what the artist has produced and relate it to its context including the traditions and conventions which shaped it. This, as we shall see later, is really the key aim of a critical appreciation of the Arts. See also Strawson, 1974, p. 185.

The story of Daedalus and Icarus

Daedalus and Icarus, of course, were the father and son who made themselves wings of feathers and wax in order to escape from imprisonment on a Mediterranean island. Icarus flew too near the sun, the wax melted and he fell into the sea and drowned.

Here we have a very short story! Well – at least – that is the *end* of a story. And told like that, in a few very simple sentences, it might seem that there is little to comment upon. Indeed, readers may not even be sure what their reaction to it should be. Even from this, then, we can begin to see that successful story-telling, and the ability to invest the story with a significance beyond the basic narrative, depends on the teller controlling a number of issues. And that is partly where the artistry of story-telling comes from. For example, there is an appeal, a subtle pressure, at the start of the story as presented above in the words 'of course'. They draw the reader into working with the teller by calling on memory of similar stories almost inevitably learnt at school, probably barely remembered and yet expected to be part of the cultural heritage of the Western world. (What effect did my version of the story have on you as you read it? Did it foster a relationship between you (as reader) and the story and/or me as teller? Did it operate as a useful shorthand to save me repeating known information or did it block the possibility to admitting that you could not remember or did not know as much about these two characters as you perhaps felt you ought?)

Further, the story as I have offered it here is begun very near to its chronological end. (How, then, does the reader who remembers very little or who never knew the wider story know what to make of it?) Information about character, motivation and previous history are all held back. What led up to this 'end', what kind of an end is it? How should the reader judge the death? What emotions should the reader feel? If we know or remember no more than is offered above, then it is not clear whether the pair in this story are heroes or villains. It is not clear what the story is about – how it should be interpreted. Is it about wilful stupidity? Is it a moral tale designed around a striking image of 'man' falling (represented by Icarus) and failing to survive in an environment belonging to – God, or the gods, or the sky? Is it about disobedience and what happens to a son who flouts his father's orders and experiences the inevitable results of over-ambition? (Are there echoes here of later Christian stories?) Is it about technological error, or does it offer an allegory which points up the dangers inherent in artistry and innovation?

Anyone unfamiliar with or unable to remember the story would begin to know what it was really about only if more details were offered. The context of the story is missing, the traditions within which the story is told are missing and the characterization and earlier fortunes of the two protagonists are missing. The form in which the story is presented is, in this case, two sentences which deliver in apparently factual terms information which cannot be accepted as 'fact'. And, in terms of style, the very simple sentence structure provides almost nothing to latch on to, except that, read aloud, the sound of the second sentence, with its falling cadence, echoes the falling of Icarus. The narrator (the person through whom the story is told) is not involved in the action and gives away neither any emotion in response to the story nor any indication of what it might mean.

In fact, the apparent simplicity and factual tone ironically belie the content. The story is myth, from the legends of Crete which (according to *The New Larousse Encyclopedia of Mythology*, 1972) were imported early into Greece and were the basis of Hellenic mythology. Myths have two major functions: to answer fundamental questions about how the world came to be, and secondly to justify an existing system and to account for traditional rites and customs. They are traditionally remodelled to reflect changes brought about by revolution or evolution, and this story naturally took on new aspects as it became adapted to continental traditions. For the Cretans the Daedalus story was part of a myth which centred for the most part round the figure of the fabulous King Minos, who, as King of Crete, was famous for the wisdom of his laws and his sense of justice. Thus the story may have been, in its original form, about the grandeur of Minos and the Cretan culture and the 'natural' punishment (by the sun) of those who did not acknowledge this. (Minos had married Pasiphae who had given him several children before Poseidon, angered by Minos, inspired her with a monstrous passion for a bull. From their union was born the Minotaur (half monster, half human). This monster, who fed exclusively on human flesh, had been imprisoned in a labyrinth constructed by Daedalus.)

Myths develop as culture spreads, however, and the Greeks fashioned these ideas into a legend to fit their own ideas and beliefs. But we actually learn the story principally through Ovid, a Roman poet whose main subject was the exploits of the Greeks and who seems to have provided us with access to the Greek interpretation. The story appeared in *Metamorphoses* VIII. (This raises questions about whose story this actually is, who is telling it and how it has come into possession of the teller.) For the Greeks, the story of Daedalus was not an explanation of the development of Cretan culture but was part of the establishment and celebration of their own values, being related to the story of their great hero Theseus, whose exploits were a recurring theme in many of their legends. It is a story of fierce contrasts. From it we learn that Daedalus had been a wicked man. Daedalus the artificer did violence to nature in trying to enter where man is not equipped to go. And yet, that too is not all the story. He was distinguished both for his cunning and his ingenuity. He was a brilliant inventor and craftsman. He invented the axe and the saw, yet he killed his nephew, a rival craftsman, and sought asylum with King Minos at Crete. Here Daedalus helped Ariadne (Minos' daughter who had fallen in love with Theseus) to enable Theseus to escape from the Labyrinth where he had been imprisoned by Minos. For this treachery King Minos had Daedalus and Icarus locked up in the Labyrinth for a while. They flew from Crete to freedom by means of wax wings invented (improvised) by Daedalus.

It is easy to misread the meaning enshrined in myths, but it seems that Icarus' death was not so much an error brought about by his being imprudent enough to fly too near the sun so that the wax melted as an inevitable fate brought about because of the character and life of Daedalus. By further development, the Ovidian tradition had it that moderation and the golden mean (*medio tutissimus ibis*) are essential to the good life. The following translation of Ovid's epigraph '*Et ignotas animum dimittit in artes*' (which is also quoted at the front of Joyce's *Portrait of the Artist as a Young Man*) shows the fall as inevitable and gives a flavour of the poetic style.

> In tedious exile now too long detain'd
> Dedalus languish'd for his native land.
> The sea forclos'd his flight; yet thus he said,
> Though earth and water in subjection laid,
> O cruel Minos, thy dominion be,
> We'll go though air; for sure the air is free.
> *Then to new arts his cunning thought applies,*
> *And to improve the work of nature tries.* (See Kenner, 1955, p. 134)

The rest you know – except that Daedalus survived, landed in Cumae, went on to Sicily and gained the favour of the King Cocalus. Minos, however, pursued Daedalus there but Cocalus refused to hand Daedalus over and instead drowned Minos in a bath. (This raises an interesting question about where a story actually ends.)

Telling this story in a particular order, then, is a means of controlling the reader's interest in and response to it. Story-telling is a fascinating art and one that professionals are beginning to use much more seriously as a means of investigating their practice. However, story-telling is often treated in professional contexts as a useful but relatively simple matter. This would suggest that professionals need to understand better the disciplines involved and be more aware of its real potential as a professional vehicle.

The myth of Daedalus and Icarus has captured the interest of Western civilization and has become a reference point for a number of other pieces of art and art forms which have appeared in a number of countries. For example, in Rome at the Villa Albani is an (undated) antique bas-relief of Daedalus and Icarus showing the boy being fitted with huge wings (see *The New Larousse Encyclopedia of Mythology*, 1972, p. 197). It was, as we shall see, of interest to the Dutch painter Bruegel in the sixteenth century, and in the twentieth century it figures in the Auden poem. But James Joyce too makes deliberate reference to it, using Daedalus as the surname for his flawed hero in his lyrical novel *A Portrait of the Artist as a Young Man* (first published in 1916). This novel, which there is no space here to consider in detail, yields much to the reader who seeks to appreciate it by the means being illustrated in relation to the myth, the painting and the poem, and which are offered in detail in the second part of this chapter. Such an appreciation would reveal the interwoven images and themes of which the novel is made up and the essential moral ambivalence of the work, and why it is not entirely clear how seriously the reader should take Stephen Daedalus (who in wishing to be an artist also seeks to improve the work of nature rather than appreciating it). In all these examples, the reader (or audience) is expected to respond with recognition and knowledge to the original myth and the maker is using it to enrich and extend *his* own artefact by such references, as we shall now see in more detail. (It will have been noted that all these are male artists and this point is extended later.)

Bruegel the Elder's *Landscape and the Fall of Icarus*

It is not entirely clear when this picture (see Plate 6.1) was painted, and there is some dispute about the authorship. But it is believed to be by Pieter Bruegel and to have been painted either about 1558, or about 1568, the year before Bruegel's death. It is currently in the Musées Royaux des Beaux-Arts, Brussels, with a smaller version in the D. M. van Buuren collection in New York. The Dutch more or less invented 'landscape painting'. This is a picture of an Italian landscape in which is placed the climax of a Greek myth, and it is painted by a Flemish painter who had travelled in Italy (but never to Greece) and who was working at the height of a terrible crisis in visual art. (The coming of Protestantism made the traditional Christian subjects of Madonna and Child no longer acceptable, to the point where painters were robbed of their main source of subject matter.) In fact this is the only painting by Bruegel on a classical theme, but he did produce a number of paintings on quite different subjects which also acted a parables. None of his work has a directly religious content.

In this oil painting the named subject is barely visible in the corner of the fairly large canvas (which measures twenty-nine inches by just over forty-four inches). All that we see of Icarus,

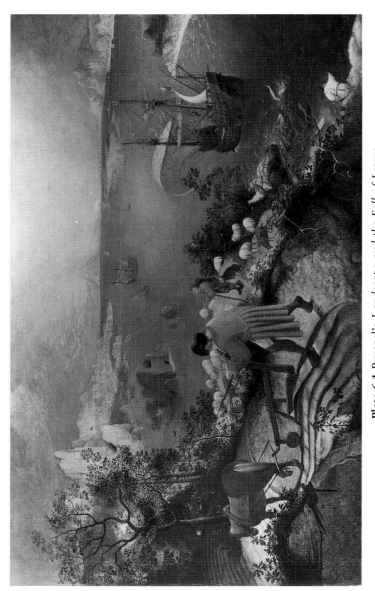

Plate 6.1 Bruegel's *Landscape and the Fall of Icarus*

on the right hand lower side of the picture, is two legs and feet disappearing into the sea – in what seems to be a final kick to maintain life. Throughout the rest of the painting much else is happening. We are above, overlooking the scene – and are thus detached from it. Our eye is drawn first to the ploughman who is the nearest and largest figure and whose bright red shirt is a sharp contrast to the rest of the colours of the scene. A painter works by controlling (consciously or sub-consciously) line, colour, tone, texture and most of all, here, by means of composition. This ensures that we become aware of a number of elements in the painting (though not, of course, necessarily in the *order* described below).

From the ploughman the eye is drawn by the light on the water, out to the wide and empty sweep of sea towards a horizon near which is a distant town. The sea and the distant town are catching the low light of the dying sun, which, having done its damage to Icarus' wings is now going down behind the sea. Its beams also catch the ploughman and the legs of Icarus, but much of the rest of the picture is, by contrast, in subdued tones as befits an evening scene, and some, as we shall see, is even darker. Turning back to the human interest (it is very clear why the title of the painting puts the landscape first), we realize that in the foreground are not one but three people: the ploughman, a shepherd and a fisherman. But all have their backs to Icarus and are looking away from him. In the middle ground to the right is what the eye interprets as a large ship with billowing sails which is also already beyond Icarus and is being blown rapidly further from him. We note all this with unemotional sympathy resulting from our distance from it and height above it.

The smaller version of this painting, held in New York, has Daedalus in shadowy form in the sky. It is lacking in the Brussels version, but may have been there too, originally, since it has been at some time transferred from panel to canvas. With him or without, the picture still says the same: life goes on. Yet death is there too, and not only in the figure of Icarus. As the eye travels round the picture (a response contrived by the painter's composition and particularly the lines depicting the ridges of the ploughed land at the very front of the picture), it eventually picks out under the darkness of some trees, a dead body. I had looked at reproductions of the picture a number of times before I saw it. And yet the ploughman's horse, plodding downhill takes us directly to the white blob of the cadaver's face. The Italian landscape setting with its wide sweep of sea and sky, its islands and a distant harbour may dominate the scene, but the painting is clearly not merely an excuse for a landscape. We know that other of his paintings depict famous proverbs and *Landscape and the Fall of Icarus* seems to be in tune with the original Ovidian interpretation, and also at one with a German proverb of Bruegel's time: 'no plough is stopped for the sake of a dying man' (see Stechow, 1990, p. 50). Indeed, Bruegel seems to have adhered in all but one point to the original Ovid, which Stechow (1990, p. 50) translates as:

> [Beneath], someone catching fish with his tremulous rod,
> The shepherd leaning on his crook, or the ploughman on his handle,
> Saw them and wondered how they could take to the air
> And thought they must be gods. Already, on the left,
> They passed by Samos, Juno's isle, and by Delos and Paros;
> And on the right, by Labinthos and Calymne, fruitful in honey . . .

Bruegel makes the ploughman and fisherman concentrate on their work. They look down. Only the shepherd looks up – but even then he is turned away from Icarus (perhaps towards the now missing Daedalus). Bruegel has, too, in several senses deliberately gone beyond the traditions of the art of the time. He has turned to myth rather than sacred subject. He has fused landscape with story, focusing on two ideas not one, and brought Italian and Greek ideas together in ways not done before. He has thus made new connections and enabled us to see an old story anew.

This painting was seen, apparently in the 1930s, by W. H. Auden, in Brussels where it still hangs. (The resulting poem is included in a section of poems written between 1933 and 1938). He in his turn, using a different art form, enables us to see the painting anew and to see in it a rather more modern version of its meaning. His response to Bruegel's work was as follows.

W. H. Auden's *Musée des Beaux Arts*

> About suffering they were never wrong,
> The Old Masters: how well they understood
> Its human position; how it takes place

While someone else is eating or opening a window or just
    walking dully along;
How, when the aged are reverently, passionately waiting
For the miraculous birth, there always must be
Children who did not specially want it to happen, skating
On a pond at the edge of the wood:
They never forgot
That even the dreadful martyrdom must run its course
Anyhow in a corner, some untidy spot
Where the dogs go on with their doggy life and the torturer's horse
Scratches its innocent behind on a tree.

In Brueghel's *Icarus*, for instance: how everything turns away
Quite leisurely from the disaster; the ploughman may
Have heard the splash, the forsaken cry,
But for him it was not an important failure; the sun shone
As it had to on the white legs disappearing into the green
Water; and the expensive delicate ship that must have seen
Something amazing, a boy falling out of the sky,
Had somewhere to get to and sailed calmly on.

                                        (Auden, 1968, pp. 123–124)

Auden's poem whose title is the only means of our understanding
its context, presents us with very little of what he has physically
seen as he stood in the gallery where Bruegel's painting hangs, but
rather it offers us what he has *understood* (seen with his mind's
eye) as a result of his physical seeing.

The poem is divided into two parts and in that sense operates
rather like a sonnet, although it is not one. The first thirteen lines
offer us the philosophical ideas of the poem, which arise from
looking at some (unnamed) paintings of (unnamed) Old Masters.
These paintings are seen to comment on the inevitability of suffering, its agony and how it takes place, unrecognized, in a corner,
while the rest of the world goes on with its (rather dull and fairly
hopeless) life. The second part focuses in detail on Bruegel's painting, as an example of this, and points out elements of it in ways
that make us see it again.

In the first section Auden illustrates how the Old Masters (the
great painters, who inevitably have had a moral dimension to their
work) contrast the often secret and usually unrecognized agony of
human suffering with the dull ordinariness of other human life
which goes on (and must go on) oblivious of it. He cites everyday
actions in a long fourth line which seems to portray their end-

lessness and which is all the more successful because the previous two lines are also broken in the middle by punctuation and thus provide even shorter units of speech. He startles the reader by depicting the aged reverently waiting for 'the miraculous birth' (rather than death) and notes how this no doubt is (he uses the present tense tellingly) in contrast to the unawareness of children at play. He depicts the aged as always aware ('they never forgot' – and we are in suspense until the next line which is highlighted because of this) that the 'dreadful martyrdom' (perhaps even just the bad bits of 'life') must happen in a corner which animals make dirty and where the *innocent* horse whose job is usually to bear a *cruel* man (again the suspense of the end of a line in the middle of the meaning) scratches its behind on a tree. And all this is offered in a quiet and casual, conversational tone of one already in converse informally with a fellow visitor to the gallery. This relaxed sense is added to by the loose and free rhythm which echoes the sound of ordinary speech, but which is held together by a barely audible, yet central, and very strict rhyme scheme.

In contrast to the first part of the poem, is the shortened second section which, rather as in a sonnet, follows the longer first section and reinforces the argument by reference to a specific example. Here we turn to the specifics of the Bruegel painting, which is named in the first line. He points out the 'leisurely' turning away of 'everything' from the disaster. Here he is describing the *speed* not the *occupations* of those involved. And again here he uses, to create tension in the first two lines, the caesura (the pause in the middle of the line – which is a device common to classical, medieval and renaissance poetry and is thus appropriate to the subject matter). And this prepares for the third line where the sound of the drama is created by the syntax, so that we hear that 'the ploughman may (new line) have heard the splash' (short moment of dramatic action) and 'the forsaken cry'. (Here we have an even shorter phrase, made final by the end of the line coinciding with the end of the sentence and at the same time rendered rather pathetic by the brevity of the word 'cry' which almost sounds as if it is being snatched away by the wind and which has little hope of being heard at a distance). Indeed, Auden seems here to be creating for us a set of sympathetic emotions of a kind which the painter distanced us from!

The poem goes on to say that for the ploughman, the fall of

Icarus was 'not an important failure' and the word 'failure' comes as a more blatant statement of moral judgement than any we have heard so far, though Auden is not interested in *whose* failure it is. Even the sun carried on its job. Fate being in control, it 'shone [end of line] As it had to [this increased the sense of inevitability] on the white legs disappearing into the green [end of line] Water;' (here we have the elongated fall again captured by the syntax and lay-out). The delightful, strange and contrasted image of the 'expensive delicate ship', as an unexpectedly appropriate way of describing a huge wooden structure, captures perfectly the realistic and yet romantic and elegant aura of the large and powerful and yet fragile craft which Bruegel painted. We realize through these adjectives that its delicate nature is a reminder of man's. (The image partly reminds us of its thin masts and rigging and partly warns that despite its power it would be helpless, as Icarus has been, against nature's onslaught.) And the ship (now standing as a symbol for all the souls on it) 'saw something amazing, a boy falling out of the sky', and even then does not turn to investigate but, having somewhere to get to, 'sailed calmly on' – and again the inevitability of it all, of life going on despite tragedy, comes through. But this poem was written in between two World Wars, and so this whole subject matter of suffering and life going on had for contemporary readers a less comfortable and yet more encouraging note about it than can be the case for a reader in a relatively safer world.

What we have been involved in here is critical appreciation of examples from the Arts. We have looked at each as a whole, but have noticed some details within that whole and responded to the writer's, painter's and poet's vision while recognizing the means by which they present it. To some extent this involves interpretation rather than a straight 'summary' of the work. The whole point of the Arts is that they say things in ways that cannot be bettered or even equalled, so that a summary is always inferior to the original, and will always introduce a particular way of seeing it. However, what has been offered is a beginning in 'seeing' these pieces of art. It is not claimed to be the only possible reading of them. Indeed, the reader is warmly invited to consider these works much more carefully than this critique does and then to form his or her own view. But neither do these comments invalidate what has been offered. Art is multi-dimensional. It expresses complexities. It yields to a range of interpretations, any one of which is valid as long as it can be illustrated in detail by honest and accurate reference to the piece of art *as a whole*.

Such an approach to appreciation, as illustrated above (which consists essentially of a recognition and a presentation of what is there) is also available to professional practitioners for use in recognizing, responding to and understanding the art of their professional work, and here too, it is being argued, a holistic approach needs to be taken. In order to benefit from the possibilities of this, however, practitioners need to consider in more detail the language and ideas involved in appreciation.

Responding to artistry: the language of appreciation

This section will look in turn at concepts (and therefore language) which are the central means of recognizing and responding to (thinking and writing about) the Arts, and which by this token are also of interest to practitioners seeking to appreciate their practice. By reference to the above critiques which focused on the Daedalus and Icarus theme, firstly are considered some key critical ideas (together with their associated language) which are common across all the Arts and secondly some language useful for appreciating (reading) literature and looking at paintings is offered.

The language of appreciation as common to all the Arts

The ideas in this section, then, have all been drawn upon in the above discussions of the myth, painting and poem on the Daedalus and Icarus theme. They are however all equally useful in talking of work in music, drama, film, opera, dance and the artistry of practice. In many cases, however, the apparently simple language for talking about art is in fact full of subtle but important divisions and distinctions which result from different ways (and fashions) of looking at different subjects within the Arts. Once understood by the critic, they are useful for appreciating (exploring meaning in and for formulating a response to) a specific work of art, and they are also a help in understanding better what is involved in critical appreciation and in the creation of works in the Arts.

Art and the maker

An artist 'makes' his or her art with a considerable degree of conscious intention so to do (though there might well be a major element of unconscious intention present too). This statement does not however exclude the existence within the artistic process of elements of chance and discovery, nor even that such elements may or may not have been preserved and extended by a 'maker' who recognizes them and intends to utilize them in the process of that creation. And in considering these matters we should not forget that in professional practice the practitioner too is a maker, who makes and works upon meanings in the professional context. The artist, depending on his or her raw materials, creates in a variety of different media. The painter uses a range of paints, brushes, and paper or canvas, vellum or plaster; the writer uses language; the professional practitioner 'makes meaning' in the professional context with clients, patients and pupils through words and actions, thoughts, emotions and motives, reasoning and judgements.

In the realm of the Arts, however, there is much more doubt than there used to be about whether the artist is in control of his or her medium or whether the medium is in control of the artist. For example, both through its inevitable limitations and in the tyranny of its traditions any medium, once chosen, inevitably imposes certain decisions upon the artist. Thus there were certain effects that Bruegel, working in the sixteenth century, would not have been able to achieve through a painted landscape even had he wished to. Some of these are about his choice of oil rather than acrylic, for example, and here we note that choice was also constrained by the traditions and times in which he worked (acrylic not having been invented). So, while there is modern scepticism about the idea that an artist is the origin and end of the meaning of a work of art, it is also important to recognize the constraints within which he or she operates. The practitioner is, knowingly or unknowingly, beset by similar constraints.

In literary studies, Barthes has argued for the 'death of the author' precisely because it is possible for the audience to value a work of art in ways that go beyond the artist's original vision. However, it could be argued that in doing so he has merely saddled the audience (reader) with more, rather than fewer responsibilities for knowing about the author and his times, in order to ensure that what is claimed as a *new* understanding is expressed appropriately so as not to misrepresent the original. What Barthes perhaps has achieved however is, importantly, to draw our attention to the multi-dimensional character of a work of art and thus also to the notion that there is no one right deciphering of it (see Barthes, 1977).

Foucault, by contrast, has argued that an author is a mere 'historical construction', because the significance and meaning of a work of art varies across time – both for other artists (as indeed, we have seen the meaning and significance of the myth of Daedalus and Icarus change) – and for audiences. Clearly it is true that the significance of a work of art for the author also varies in different historical times, and in different cultures because values and traditions of discourse change. Foucault also argues that the author is not necessarily an authority on his or her work, and reminds us that in medieval times the names of the authors of ballads, songs and stories, which were circulated by word of mouth, were quickly forgotten or never known, but that this did not affect the estimate of the artistic merit of those pieces. However, in spite of all this, 'the figure of the author remains a decisive force in contemporary culture' (see Bennett and Royle, 1995, p. 24). Bennett and Royle also suggest that 'the greatest literary texts are indeed those into which the author has most effectively vanished. The most powerful works of literature are those which suggest that they are singular, that no one else could have written them, *and yet* that their authorship is irrelevant' (Bennett and Royle, 1995, pp. 25–26). But even this does not prevent us wanting to know more about them as we study their work more deeply!

There has, thus, been a fashion recently to belittle the 'authority' of artists about their work. For example, it has been argued that to ask of artists what they *meant* or *intended* by their work is often actually impossible, for one reason or another, and in any case their reply would not necessarily provide a basis for discussing the work or an appropriate standard against which to judge it. Even where an artist can make a statement of intention, that, it is argued, would only become another creation about which various interpretations would be possible, and artists might not be entirely open about their work or as astute about the meaning and value of it as another critic might be.

None the less, wherever it is possible to know who the author is or was and something about him or her, and therefore to be aware

this says something about the culture and values of the times and of the artists. By contrast, a poststructuralist or deconstructive reading of a work of art might also trace the dispersal or dissolution of the audience's identity, which is endemic to the act of response to art. Is the role of the audience determined by the artistic object or vice versa? But is a work of art really only to be seen as 'incomplete', ready to be remade by every new response? Might not both of these views exist side by side – so that a faithful response to the artist's vision and an individual one are both required, and both are subjected to judgement by the critical community? And might not these ideas be echoed in the appreciation of the artistry of professional practice?

The relationship of form and content in the Arts

One of the most commonly held principles in the Arts is that the form or structure of the work of art should be peculiarly appropriate in some way to the content – even that there should be some sort of unity or harmony between form and content. It is thus useful to determine something of the themes (motifs) of the work where appropriate, and where possible simultaneously, to recognize how the composition supports this as part of the meaning. Thus, the way something is said should normally be considered as part of what is being said (even if the artist is deliberately or disastrously flouting this notion, as for example in Hardy's poem *Drummer Hodge,* which captures the sadly unceremonious throwing of Hodge into his rough grave by means of verses whose inappropriate sound, when read aloud, is more like a happy dance tune). Thus, for example, we saw how in the myth of Daedalus and Icarus, as I presented it, the story form and structure through which it was told, directly controlled, made specific and limited the meaning of the events for the reader.

In Bruegel's painting too, the composition is designed to enable us to appreciate the moment of Icarus' death in a particular way. The placing of his sinking legs, the ship, the ploughman, shepherd and fisherman make a comment about life going on in spite of death which is so clear that those who rarely look at a painting find no trouble in understanding it. And the lines of the ploughed land, once observed, also seem clearly designed to lead us to see the body beneath the trees, and, by taking us on round the picture, link this separate tragedy back up to the Icarus story and thus perhaps to popular sayings about death and the continuance of life. Here again then, we cannot respond to the painting without recognizing that the composition is itself part of the content and meaning of this work.

Similarly, in Auden's poem, the sonnet-like form provides a perfect structure within which to explore a general idea in terms of a specific example. The first stanza, which is rather like an octave but longer, offers a broad comment about suffering, which is then grounded in a specific picture found in the second stanza, which is like a sestet only longer. There is too a kind of irony in the fact that unlike most sonnets, the 'picture' presented to the reader in the second part of the poem is more than just figurative, it is a 'real' painting – but not of a real person.

This in turn points up the importance (in some poems) of the *gap* between stanzas. Where there are two parts to a poem, as here, the gap often acts as a hinge, allowing the poem to be 'opened up'. Where there are more verses, stanzas or sections, they often indicate that a change has taken place during the 'interval' between them – that some new action has taken place off-stage as it were, between one and the next. (John Donne's skittishly serious poem *The Flea* is a perfect example of this. Here, each verse carries the voice of a lover wooing a lady and contriving his arguments for her to yield to him by responding to her reactions to a crisis which is going on simultaneously – of her first discovering and then later killing a flea. In fact, ironically, the poem is as much about the speciousness of the lover's arguments as about the flea and the woman. To fail to recognize the three-act shape of the poem and how the hopeful lover is using *her implied actions* in deploying *his* arguments, is to miss half the fun and most of the seriousness of the poem.)

Similarly, it is important to attend to any framing devices the artist uses, looking closely too at the beginning and the end of any art which has a chronological element, and the use of suspense. These devices provide ways of controlling information that the artist offers the audience, thus shaping audience perception of the meaning and their response to the overall work. By these means we are introduced to (via titles and other 'peritexts'), guided through (by means of compositional devices) and cut off from (by frames and endings) the content contained within a work of art. For example, in the version of the myth which I offered, we broke into the story near its tragic climax, and the story was cut off long before its chronological end, which was offered later. (But where do stories begin and end? For a detailed exploration of the issues related to this, see Bennett and Royle, 1995.) In Bruegel's picture we are presented (on a canvas of specific dimensions only) with a frozen moment at the very climax of a known story and this is explored in broader human terms, the bystanders getting (literally) larger parts than the protagonist whose name and actions offered in the painting's title, provide a means of 'framing' our understanding of it. And in Auden's poem the title plays a vital role in supplying us with information not available elsewhere.

We can see in these examples, then, that in appreciating art, to tease content and form apart and to analyse them separately without due regard to this wholeness is, in a sense, both to fail to understand what they are about and to disrupt the essential integrity of art. To respond to meaning in art, to reach the heart of the experience it offers, is to respond to form and content *together*.

Recognizing and responding to style
It is also useful, having perhaps discovered something of what the artist is trying to say and of the way it demands to be expressed, to be able to recognize and respond to the *means* by which that artist achieves the shaping of form to suit content. In different art forms, of course, different media are used. Thus the painter chooses amongst tempera, oil, watercolour, acrylic, pastel, gouache, ink, charcoal, pencil and various printing materials together with a variety of means of applying these to a variety of surfaces, while the range of a writer's materials is, in some ways, less varied. Further, for all such artists, style and expression are themselves shaped by the times, traditions, values and culture in which the artist lives and out of which he or she makes something new. Whatever materials are used however, and whatever traditions are influential, they are (consciously or unconsciously) deployed by the artist – in all forms of the Arts – *in ways appropriate to the meanings being created,* to produce tone (light and shade), texture and pattern, colour and shape, image and imagery, allegory and symbol, rhythm. And in shaping *these* an artist can utilize (consciously or unconsciously) juxtaposition, proportion, balance, harmony, gradation, contrast, variation, dominance.

These ideas are neither difficult nor obscure but there is no point in defining these terms in the broad context of the Arts generally because they have specific and in some cases differing meanings within different arts. Tone would be an example of this, since although it always refers to light and shade, it is used to refer to density in painting, and to vocal expression in writing. Further, the problem is not in understanding these terms (even in differing contexts), but in recognizing their use in a work whose unity has been so well crafted that form and content have almost merged. For this reason, they are focused on in the more detailed sections below. In this sense it is like professional practice, where the visible skills belie the practitioner's invisible expertise and judgement.

Reading the written word: language for appreciating literature

There are many aspects of the appreciation of literature which could be advanced as potentially helpful to professional practitioners who seek to understand their practice. These include particularly: narrative form; characterization, style and expression; figurative language; voice (and matters of comedy and tragedy); syntax and 'the performative' (doing things with words). They are each discussed below.

Narrative form

Most of our lives involve the telling of and listening to stories. We often use them to help us to understand something better. For example, we tell them to explore or explain our dreams, actions, history, motives, aspirations; and we read and hear them in newspapers, books, television, radio, films. Conflicting stories often lead to disagreements and even wars. For the professional, story-telling and hearing has some particularly important roles to play in helping us to understand our clients and in helping us to explore our own practice. These are stories that we tell and hear, but which, at the same time we are also part of. And we learn early in professional practice, if not in our early life, that there is always more than one version of a story. This, of course can be turned to positive use in trying to understand something through a story. And one of the things that we can learn to understand better is the art of story-telling itself. The following looks at two main aspects of narrative: at those matters related to its linearity (the order of events presented in the story), and those elements concerned with the relationship between the teller and the listener or reader.

Narrative form: linearity
The simplest way to define narrative is a series of events in a specific order – usually having a beginning, middle and end. The shaping of narrative is, as we have already seen, an important consideration in story-telling, whether the story be told in poetry, prose or drama form. And this shaping is directly related to time. Often, for a variety of reasons, the story jumps about in time sequence. This also mirrors what happens when we start to tell a story that we have not previously thought through, because the memory does not always help us to 'remember' sequences in chronological order and we move temporally backwards and forwards in asides and diversions as we remember more. But even when we are at the point of relating a story in straight chronological order, that temporal sequencing of events is not the whole story. What also matters is the relationship (or not) between two events and whether one was caused by the other or was in some other way connected to it. (The relationships of events in the Daedalus myth are adjusted by different authors by means of different structuring of the story and this causes the story to carry a different emphasis.) The logical or causal connections between events in a story are a fundamental aspect of all narratives. By the same token, where the story starts and ends is significant (as we have already seen in my own version of the Daedalus myth) and in addition, the kind of story being told and the kind of suspense available to the teller depends on whether the reader or audience knows from the start what the end will be. Often a narrative moves from a stable state, through a disturbance and back to a new stability, so that the end becomes the main place for revelation and understanding, thus satisfying the reader's desire to know. This has led readers to become accustomed to look to the end for 'answers'. But, of course there are often no answers in life and modern narratives recognize this by providing unresolved endings.

There is a sense too in which a story is made up of both the events *and* the telling of those events. Thus, the actions which are said to have occurred interact with, but can to some extent be teased apart from, the way in which they are told (including the organization of the narrative). Many nineteenth and twentieth century British and American novelists have experimented with these two elements and make the reader work at relating them or disentangling one or other, or both. Famous examples include *Wuthering Heights* which has a meticulously worked out, complex narrative structure which moves about in time but which is not always obvious on surface reading. Other examples are the novels of Joseph Conrad, of Henry James and of Alain Robb-Grillet. Most postmodernist texts (for example the novels of Umberto Eco) find ways of challenging the expectations associated with these ideas, as a means of shaking the reader out of previous assumptions about narrative.

Narrative form: relationships between teller and listener

Who the teller is, and what his or her relationship is to the story and to the listeners, also provide some interesting means by which narrative can be considered. For example, it is important in responding fully to a story for the reader to consider whether it is told in the first or third person, is told by someone inside or outside the events, whether the teller is a reliable or doubtful witness, is omniscient about or confined to a very narrow view of events and characters, and what point of view the story is told from and in what voice.

William Hildick elucidated thirteen types of narrative, and their different uses. There is more than simply a choice between biographical or autobiographical form and/or the narrator who might stand to one side. There is, combined with these, a choice of tense and of mode. For example Hildick's third type of narrative is 'the use of first person past, as if spoken' (useful, he says, for the most full characterization of the story-teller and for developing a sense of suspense). This may be compared with 'the use of the first person past, as if written' which he says is useful in presenting tragedy as it allows the presentation of planning, preparation and action by one who was involved and who can now look back with hindsight, and who is, of course, in a position to point up the morals (see Hildick, 1968, p. 52). Such a stance on the part of the writer also brings with it implications for the role of the reader; for example, in the last case, the reader is aware that the writer knows something he is not yet telling, and will be expected to wait for more information, and be told how to think about it.

The diary form is Hildick's tenth type of narrative. It has overtones of a historical document, records 'ups and downs' over a long period and allows for the combining of momentous public and significant private events and a registering of their impact. Placing diary extracts in a wider framework helps the narrative to capture the complexity of life. The orderly scrapbook (the literary version of a documentary) is his eleventh type, and interestingly he points up its 'clinical impersonality' by comparison with most others. Presumably also it is here that the collage (or, as in the work of Dos Passos, 'montage') fits. The interior monologue, stream of consciousness and 'progression d'effet' technique are all means of presenting those fleeting thoughts, impressions and emotions inside a character's head, which provide depth of characterization, flow beneath the surface of observable action and unite past and present. What Hildick calls 'string of pearls' (a series of discrete first person narratives in a third person framework) allows for all sorts of people to enter the scene and to offer further information and new perspectives.

This however is only one way of categorizing narrative technique. There are, too, various classic narrative forms, used by the teller and expected to be known and recognized by the listener. For example, classical tragedy has a shape which enables it to demonstrate the fall of a great person as inevitable. The story of Daedalus could be recounted in this mode, first building up the character and talents of Daedalus and then using a series of events through which to alert us to his folly and inevitable fall. By contrast, his story could also be told as a picaresque (a series of barely connected comic stories associated with a journey). I have long thought that this form offers great scope for writing about professional practice. Such a structure would be full of digression, suspension, aphorisms and self-reflection. In picaresque what is compelling is the very disorder which is endemic in the events we are presented with, and which is paralleled by the very presentation of those events. Also important for professionals looking at storytelling to help their work, is what Joyce called 'epiphanies' (returning light), which are moments of sudden insight which the characters have and which the reader can be led to regard and respond to in a number of ways.

Beyond this too there is the critical issue of point of view (how and from whom we learn the story). And there is much more to it than, for example, a choice between the omniscient narrator (the really efficient 'fly on the wall'), the detached observer (where the reader is held at a distance for a variety of reasons) and the biographical or autobiographical form. There is single and central 'point of view' where we learn the story directly from one narrator only and deduce other perspectives from the way he or she reacts with the world. There is double point of view where the story is told by two different narrators (of which *Wuthering Heights* is a striking but subtle example). And there is the shifting or bouncing viewpoint offering a range of narrators (which leaves the reader to make a judgement). Allied to all this is the use of psychological as opposed to chronological time sequences and stories that create their own special time or whole history. In a novel whose chronology is deliberately disjointed in order to juxtapose events which are not actually related in time, the novelist often uses an event or sound (like a huge gun firing once) which is heard by different groups of people each in their own 'time capsule' incident. This is a means of anchoring the chronological relationship of events. (It was a favourite technique of Conrad, for example.) Such a mixing of chronological and psychological time allows for an amalgam of perception, memory, speculation.

Beyond these however there are also interesting issues of coincidence, relevance and contingency for the story-teller to juxtapose. For example, in a fast moving thriller a quick 'shot' of a man standing in the mist will have relevance for later (and the reader knows in advance that it will). This, like coincidence, can often produce a strong reaction in an audience. Yet for novelists like Iris Murdoch (who is a describer rather than an explainer) life is full of contingencies – whimsical, fey, outrageous and frankly unbelievable things that happen all at the same time but whose coincidence does not have significance. (Postmodernists of course take off from this point, considering everything to be merely contingent!)

Novelists are often also aware that a jump of even only one generation would mean deep differences of culture and that the cultural style of a society is expressed in the most ephemeral of its products (fashions in dress, life-style and so on). The significance to novelists of cultural issues is one reason why some people thought that the novel would die – for want of a clear fabric of social manners to provide it with a reference point. What novelists can assume about their readers today in respect of commonly shared knowledge, values and cultural heritage is much less than in the past. Novelists too have to choose between accuracy of description and intellectual complexity conveyed in imagery – between authenticity and interpretation.

But for all the importance of narrative form, many read a story mainly for its characters. They provide the fascination. We have strong emotional responses to them. They are the focus of life in literature. In our response to the fictional characters of literature we learn more about ourselves. If the reader does not relate to some of the characters in a story in some clear way (even if that includes judging them harshly), the story will never be successful.

Characterization

Although there is some debate about whether plot or character is more central to the success of literature, they are of course closely related, character often determining incidents, and incidents illustrating character. (Thus the character of Daedalus led to his devising the fateful wings of wax, and that of Icarus led to his flying too near the sun.) Setting too can reflect character. For example, the short stories of James Joyce in *The Dubliners* are gems of controlled poetic brevity in the way they portray character through setting, and this is particularly so in the one called 'A Painful Case' (see Joyce, 1965 [1914]).

Our memory of a story is often more of character than plot, and many famous characters from well-known stories have become part of our everyday language (Oedipus, Malaprop, Romeo, Scrooge). But of course they are fictional. What does it mean then to discuss them as if they are real? And how do story-tellers make them real, vivid and life-like? Part of the answer lies in the ability to make them plausible (to create believable names and gradually to reveal them as behaving in ways the reader recognizes as life-like). Partly too it depends upon creating a sense of complexity, presenting the character in such a way as to reveal a number of different characteristics which may well be contradictory, making the character unpredictable to a degree, implying a complexity of motives and emotions. But there also needs to be, as part of this, a sense of individual and particular identity of the character. Thus, as Bennett and Royle point out, this ' "life-likeness" appears to involve both multiplicity and unity at the same time' (Bennett and Royle, 1995, p. 51). This 'realist' approach to characterization is based upon a notion that the character is (at root) modelled on a real person. However, we also know that life sometimes seems to copy fiction and that truth is stranger than fiction. Indeed, the word 'person' goes back to the Latin 'persona' or mask or disguise, while 'character' means both a letter and a sign (an engraved mark) as well as a person's title and distinguishing mark.

The realist novel, then, relies on the idea that a person is complex but also a particular identity – in Bennett and Royle's terms 'a complex but unified whole'. As they note too, the realist novel also relies upon the familiar philosophical notion that people are made up of an inside (mind, soul, self) and an outside (body, face, and other external features) (Bennett and Royle, 1995, p. 53). In the nineteenth century the 'inside' tended to be described as 'spiritual life', while in the twentieth it is more often associated with the subconscious. And along with these notions goes the idea of the difficulty of really knowing someone – including ourselves. The notion that the inner life is hidden and needs to be inferred from outer appearances is clearly dangerous since they are often apparently in opposition, and we know full well that appearances can be deceptive. Indeed, ideas about, and the unmasking of deception, hypocrisy and disguise lie at the heart of many stories, while concerns about true identity, and the role of the 'mask' are also often explored in literature. And in the exploration of fictional characters, the reader may also safely consider his or her own. This identifying with fictional characters, then, is both dangerous and yet inevitable if literature is to be successful. Again we have ideas, also important for practitioners, that both surface and submerged characteristics are significant.

Another important dimension in narrative is the language chosen by the story-teller, which should convey the experience being presented clearly and efficiently and also appropriately. Most obvious in this catalogue is figurative language, but the writer and reader also need to take account of other key elements of style and expression, like register, dialect, syntax, the tone (neutral, sarcastic, satiric, ironic, dramatic) and the voice.

Style and expression: figurative language
Literary language is often considered as deviating from or distorting ordinary language. And, indeed, literary texts are characterized by figures of speech and these are specifically different from the language of day-to-day discourse. The point about figures of

speech is that they deviate from more literal expression. Thus, for example, hyperbole (over-exaggeration for the sake of effect); metaphor, (where one thing is likened to another); metonomy (where one thing is talked about by reference to something associated with it); and anthropomorphism (where animals are given human characteristics), or animism (where non-human things are referred to as if human) are all considered literary devices for creating new images. However most daily discourse is also littered with them! But then they are often employed without any deliberate intention. Indeed, they are often 'dead metaphors', whose constant usage has removed all impact and rendered them worn-out.

It is also important to note that the term 'image', especially as used in place of the term 'figurative language', is both useful and dangerous. It can be misleading since figurative language does not always create a picture. However, the term image is often used particularly in discussing poetry. This is because one of the chief distinctions between poetry and prose is that in prose we follow a reasoned argument and can use the tools of grammar and syntax to analyse and illustrate relationships (although this does not prevent the prose writer using all the techniques which we normally associate with poetry – even including rhyme), whereas in poetry we are immersed in a flow of images which we explore and which evoke associations and memories, thus enabling us to share the poet's experiences and feelings and remake them for ourselves. (This is why any summary of a poem will never do it justice.)

In literary criticism (or appreciation) a central question is: what is the apparently intended and the actual effect of figurative language? What is the point of it and how does it work? In successful texts it is more than merely decorative. Further, it is not always as simple as it looks.

Consider for example, the phrase we noted in the Auden poem – the 'expensive delicate ship', which does not turn back to rescue Icarus. Figures of speech may appear direct and yet they often contain elements of the elusive – they carry some ambiguity – because they recast distinctions between the real and the imagined, the literal and the figurative, the image and the word. And they fuse ideas together, leaving no trace of the join. No ship could really be delicate, or it would not survive in the sea, yet Bruegel's ship looks delicate because of its fragile looking masts. But is it also that it has been *painted* delicately? So is this a subtle reminder that the ship is not *real* in several senses (being a painting of a myth, and yet in the landscape tradition of Bruegel's time, needing to seem realistic)? And why expensive? Presumably this tells us more about the people on board. Delicate and expensive do not normally fit together in relation to a ship. Yet in some ways they do. To some extent figures of speech deal in illusion since they have a potential for hallucinatory effects like *trompe l'oeil* in painting, and they therefore need to be treated with caution. They do not however always heighten the sense of the concrete. Sometimes they make comparisons with something less visible or imaginable, by making links that do not appeal to the senses but to the mind. But whatever their make-up, they can heighten emotion, provide clues about how characters think, or sharpen meaning by introducing complexity of thought, often harnessing one idea with another unusual one so that the reader is prompted to explore the thought further. In other words, they enable us to see beneath the surface – to see what is either deliberately or unconsciously invisible, to unearth assumptions, beliefs and theories. They are a perfect vehicle for conveying uncertainty too. And all this is why figurative language for capturing professional practice is so useful.

The sound of words is also important, not only in poetry but in prose, its success depending on its being used for more than mere decoration. Examples include: anaphora (repetition), alliteration (repetition of the first letter of a series of words), assonance (repetition of internal vowel sounds across a number of words), rhyme, rhythm, cadence (the overall sound of a musical phrase) and onomatopoeia (where a word's sound mimics the thing it describes). These are all means of holding together ideas, of creating expectations in a reader (which may or may not be fulfilled), or of creating the sound of the external world being described or of the internal world of a character. An example would be the much repeated 'o' sound, with its rather mournful moan which characterizes the early lines of the Auden poem and which finds some echoes in the second stanza too. A second example from the same poem would be the way the poet arranges the 'splash, the forsaken cry', so that the word 'cry' seems to fade away and be lost as the new line and new long sentence begin (but is ironically echoed in the word 'sky' later). This has all the more impact because that 'i' sound of these two words is quite alien to all the other rhymes in the poem which are based on more open vowel sounds thus: wrong / understood / place / along / waiting / be / skating / wood / forgot / course / spot / horse / tree / away / may / (*cry*) / shone / green / seen / (*sky*) / on. This is far from a casual rhyme scheme and does much to hold the rather conversational structure of the poem together.

Such figurative language, then, gives life to texts and startles the reader into new attention and thought. It is therefore important while reading to work out how the figurative language is generated and the ways in which it disturbs the text.

The matter of symbolism, too, must be mentioned. This enables an author to link the details of character or action to a wider values system so that the reader is led to compare the happenings at one level with (for example) their historical or mythological parallels. Here, the meaning made out of the Daedalus story by first the Cretans, then the Greeks and the Romans and then Auden are obvious examples. But again, the success of this depends on a common body of knowledge (like Christianity, classical mythology or romanticism – or even other famous stories or pictorial symbols). (For example, Frank Norris' *The Octopus* charts in detail and examines the social consequences of the railway's developing tentacles as they strangle the wheat belt of North America.) By comparison with a main symbol, a theme is an illustration of ideas and concepts that occur within the novel, and a motif is an elaboration of this, and runs throughout the work as a whole.

Style and expression (words and voice)

It is quite possible for those who have become familiar with an author's writing to recognize that writer's style, in the same way as we recognize a voice and what is being said as specific to a speaker we cannot see (although this analogy cannot be carried too far). Such recognition is usually based less upon content than upon vocabulary, favourite grammatical and syntactical patterns and the sound created by these patterns, as well as typical images or typical ways of creating images, and typical tone of voice. But this is not the same as saying that there is such a thing as, for example, 'the language of poetry', meaning that there is a language fit only for poetic use, while others are not. On the other hand a successful poet often seems to be taking the words a reader might use and using them to greater effect. All poets (and other literary writers) are at once conservers of language and explorers of it. Their job

involves surprising us into a new attention to the apparently familiar in terms of language – figurative language as well as grammar
and syntax. We looked at this in the Auden poem when we considered how Auden contrived the casual conversational voice of the
poem by means of the way the sentence structure over-runs the
ends of lines so that the punctuation provides one series of pauses
which are slightly disrupted by (or contrapuntal with) the pauses
inevitably caused by the line end (because the eye has to move back
to the new line before resuming reading).

Any piece of writing has a voice. A useful critical term here is
'tone'. Here the light and shade of vocal expression is recognized.
Even where some writing is deliberately level and neutral in tone
this is an important observation, and where used in something
accorded the term 'literature' should in some way relate to content,
intention, meaning. A poet who recreates experience through
words, images, sounds, tries also to communicate a mood, which
that experience originally generated. However, a writer can exercise discipline and choice about this as about all else, and so it is
dangerous to assume a too close connection between tone of voice
and writer, or tone and experience, as if the writer 'could not help
the tone'. Rather, since a poem, for example, is a *re*-creation of
experience, it may have been shaped in tone to emphasize or suppress some emotions. In the novel to some extent, and in drama
particularly, voice is an important part of characterization. And of
course the notion of voice is present within the types of narrative
discussed above (the first person present, for example, used in a
novel or poem, speaks out of the text directly to us). Indeed, the
voice of much literature is conversational, and this too lends 'realism' to the text. Further, there is usually an interesting distinction
between the 'I' of the narrator (the persona adopted by the author)
and the real author. There are thus sometimes two voices even in
a deceptively simple seeming narration, and one (usually the 'real'
author) is often phantom-like. Recently too there has been an
emphasis on literature as a place where we especially hear multiple
voices (either many different ones or many different voices within
one person).

It is, of course, impossible to do justice to the complexities of
recognition and response to all kinds of literary texts, and the
above has therefore offered only a range of most common ideas
about narrative prose and poetry. The following seeks to widen

the examples by offering some very brief ideas about appreciating paintings. These might be of use to practitioners who are presenting a portrait (in words) of their practice, or who are providing a critique of such a portrait.

Looking at paintings: the language of appreciating visual art

This inevitably brief section seeks merely to highlight some key language which is useful for considering paintings and which has not already been discussed above. Here, key words are in bold type. I acknowledge the influence, here, of Armstrong (1996), Kent (1995), Piper (1981), Ranson (1994) and Richardson (1997). As will be quickly clear, because the ideas presented below are available to artists to create a unity in a painting, there is no one right or logical order in which to present or consider them, and indeed, in responding to a painting it is most important to look at the relationships among them, and between them and the subject matter. Further, since some of this is a matter of personal 'vision', readers may well wish to consider reorganizing these ideas for their own use, perhaps depending on the kind of painting they are interested in or the kind of portrait of professional practice they may wish to create. They have been presented here in relation to the Bruegel painting (hence the term canvas is used where for other paintings a quite different base may be appropriate).

Many of the following matters could be grouped under the main heading **composition** (which itself is a metaphor, of course). They are the elements (or some of them) that a painter (consciously or unconsciously, deliberately or intuitively) arranges in a picture and that a viewer recognizes and responds to. They all work together to make meaning in the painting, so that every ingredient – for example the size and placement of figures, tone, colour, brushwork – plays its part and altering one alters the overall meaning. A balanced composition affects us differently from a chaotically tangled one. Ranson (1994), in discussing what he calls 'distilling the scene' (capturing in it an amalgam of both the 'facts' of the scene and the emotions of the artist as he sees it) points out that seven component parts of a painting are: shape, size, line, direction (of lines and shapes), colour, value and texture, and that the eight most important principles of design are: balance (later discussed as symmetry), harmony (elements which are similar to each other), gradation (a gradual change from one thing to another), contrast (an abrupt change), variation and alternation (two ways of repeating yourself in a painting in terms of size, shape, colour), dominance (one unit being emphasized above all others) and unity (the painting needing to 'lock together rather than being merely a collection of several bits') (Ranson, 1994, p. 47). In principle then, as Kent points out, 'a picture is successful when every detail falls into place and each element – light, tone, colour, texture, form and spacing – helps create a clear and lucid image' (see Kent, 1995, p. 10). In such a way is good professional practice successful and the purpose of a professional portrait is to reveal the elements which have combined into its unity. The following attempts to look at some of this in more detail.

Scale (sheer size), though immediately obvious as an element to consider in painting, is not of course automatically an indicator of value. All that matters is that it suits the subject matter, context and the purpose of the painting. Canvases tend to be, at their larger sides, between eighteen inches and six feet. Their shape may also be significant. The canvas may be used with the longer sides horizontal (described as 'landscape') or vertical (described as 'portrait'), and the proportions of the rectangle may be altered where appropriate. Thus, for example, Bruegel's Icarus is of average size, seems to be based on the golden ratio (whose basis was a one-third to two-thirds division of a line) and is certainly not large enough to envelop the viewer. This means that the viewer can remain at a distance and retain a form of objectivity, which is important for the apparent overall intentions of the painting.

When it comes to discussing **space**, matters become more complex, not least because the painter is representing three-dimensional forms on a two-dimensional surface. Useful terms here are **'figure'** (for the key things presented, usually the hero of the story) and **'ground'** (for the areas we read as surrounding air or space or the entire set of circumstances in which the figure finds itself). Bruegel is of course playing with these notions by having the 'hero' represented only by legs and in a fairly insignificant part of the canvas. These **spatial relationships** in a painting often betray the outlook and attitudes of the painter and his culture. Orderly space which is neither cluttered nor blank suggests a serenity and optimism, whereas congestion and clutter suggests disturbance or anxiety. It might be said that but for Icarus, Bruegel's landscape has serenity. And this is true at the physical level of the composition of the painting and is one of the insights being conveyed. This is made stronger by the circular deployment of objects which we noted earlier, and which lead us round the picture (though pictures tend to be read normally from left to right in Western cultures). The key direction of lines is always significant and can be interpreted in obvious terms. In this painting the furrows already made are striking diagonal lines which unequivocally lead our eyes away from the ploughman, who looms larger at first because of where he is placed.

The scene is presented to us from a high **viewpoint** (which has associations of superiority and enables a high degree of information to be condensed into the picture, but also implies a kind of detachment and even judgement). Bruegel's painting, as we have said, tells part of a story which the viewer already knows. It depicts part of a scene and gives the impression that we are witnessing an actual event (from above). Yet at the same time we know it to be a myth and not an actual event. It thus seems appropriate that the painter provides us with a way to stay somewhat distant from the scene. The viewer of this painting is also confronted with **naturalistic space** (more or less as we perceive things normally), which makes the scene seem more believable.

But the painter has other issues to be aware of too in terms of composition. For example, total **symmetry** in a painting would not only be very boring, it would not reflect real life, where even our very bodies are asymmetrical (our faces and bodies being slightly different on each side). Paintings usually have subtle imbalances, whilst being roughly balanced in some respects, and there is a deliberate tension between these two. Extensive symmetry (of mass, weight, colour, tone, or whatever) leads to a very static picture where asymmetry is more dynamic. Imbalance can lead to greater interest, but sheer awkwardness is to be avoided.

Equally significant for painters creating the illusion of three dimensions are devices for rendering solids on a two-dimensional surface and giving them **volume** (three-dimensional space), **mass** (solidity) and **gravity** (weight). Lines and shapes on a flat surface may indicate volume and weight, but the main means of doing so is **tonal shading** which is carried out in relation to a fixed light source. In terms of **contours** it should be noted that some painters use predominantly hard, continuous lines while others use soft broken ones to denote the edges of shapes. Hard edges, of course, indicate clear focus and strong light and are useful where a separation of parts is to be emphasized, whereas soft edges convey the roundness of objects, are tactile and are seen in a light which is dimmer. They can imply fluency, integration, unity. One line which is very important to us in much of life, in many paintings, and in all landscapes, is the horizon. Where it is placed (high or low) and how it is depicted (often not as a line at all) affect the mood in terms of dramatic tension (high horizon) or ease (low horizon).

In addition to these, it is often useful to consider how **movement** is implied and represented in a painting. Movement can be seen in a number of different ways. A painter often employs devices to lead our eye from one part of a painting to another. Our eyes are drawn, for example, to track along a line, and to follow the 'thrusts and counter-thrusts of shape and line' (Piper, 1981, p. 114). In addition to this, the *subject* of a painting often includes movement which the painter catches in mid-act (and this can include implied movement, like that of the wind for example). Movement is also created by visual gradients (the increase or decrease of brightness, tilt, elongation or hue in regular sequence through pictorial space). And a painter can induce the viewer to continuous scanning of the picture by sending our eyes back and forth from one object to another, so that they jump gaps and keep seeking for similarities and analogies.

Another important aspect of painting is **light and tone**. The light that is captured in a painting – particularly in a landscape – gives it atmosphere, and by comparison darkness or dark areas are associated with evil and death. Essentially this is about not the colour but the density of the colour used – how much black or white is mixed in that colour. Half closing the eyes will exclude most of the colour and reduce a picture to its tonal values, which of course need to contrast, though how extensive such contrasts are can be controlled appropriately by the artist. Identifying the source of illumination and what it has done to the objects in the painting can be important. One result of a clear source of light is that **texture** may become significant. In discussing the texture of a painting, however, it is important to distinguish between the texture of the surface of the canvas (or other base) itself and texture as painted on that surface. Some painters of course utilize the uneven surface they are painting on or the quality of the paint and what they are using to apply it, in order to depict texture in their painting.

Naturally, a painter can also utilize **colour** as a tool of composition. How colours relate to each other visually is important. Painters play with the relationships between adjacent **hues** to make colours appear to glow or fade. How light falls on colour affects how purely that colour is seen. Painters have to work hard to produce realistic colour. And colour also can depict mood and emotion ('moody blues' being a common expression in our language) and it can operate symbolically too (blue for the Virgin Mary, white for virginity, for example).

For practitioners seeking to present and heighten a portrait of practice, the above offers both ideas and language which may help to extend their repertoire.

If this then gives some flavour of the language useful for understanding pictorial presentation, there are other matters to be attended to as part of appreciating work in the performing arts. This is particularly germane to work in professional contexts, where the practitioner is in some ways very much involved in performance. The following chapter attempts a very brief consideration of some key ideas.

7

The language of appreciation 2: watching and listening

Introduction

It is always important to have specific examples in mind when considering the language of critical appreciation. In order to discuss such a language of the performing arts, therefore, and to consider some of the language of appreciation for listening to music and watching drama and dance, it will be useful (as with the earlier discussions about literature and painting), to make reference to some works united by a theme. A theme which may well in at least some of its forms be familiar to readers is the story of Romeo and Juliet. The following discussion will therefore make references to Shakespeare's play and Tschaikovsky's *Fantasia-Overture, Romeo and Juliet*. Readers might also wish to have in mind *West Side Story* (which reshapes the story in new terms and utilizes music and dance, but which I shall not describe in detail below).

Shakespeare's *Romeo and Juliet*

A little needs to be said as a basic reminder about the tragedy of the star-crossed young lovers, which Shakespeare reshaped from an earlier poem by Arthur Brooke. (And it should be remembered that the summary below is a poor substitute for the original and is only an interpretation!) Some of it is influenced by the work of Vyvyan (1968).

   Romeo and Juliet was written for the company of Chamberlain's Men, of whom Shakespeare was a key actor, and which acted at court more often than any other theatrical company. It was probably written in the mid 1590s and was first published in 1597. It was, together with *Love's Labours Lost*, a transitional play, written when his work was already outstanding in terms of structure and thematic unity, and beginning to show 'a growing self-consciousness about language and stagecraft', and an 'ability to particularize character, made possible by the use of a freer verse movement' (Proudfoot, 1971, p. 162).

Unusually, the play is prefaced by a verse prologue (in sonnet form) in which the story – including the ending – is exactly prefigured. It is, as Barton points out, 'a play which uses antithesis as a structural principle': (love and hate; light and darkness; revelry and the tomb) (Barton, 1971, p. 229). Its first act establishes the question: in the light of the hatred between their two families (the Montagues and the Capulets) what is to be the outcome of the love between Romeo and Juliet? However, since this has already been answered in the prologue, it is clear that the play is also about why the events happen. A form of dramatic irony is therefore at work, since the audience know already (even though their source is outside the main play) much that the characters do not. Imagery abounds. White represents the forces working towards union and life; black stands for separation and death. And there is early talk of 'Fate' or 'Destiny' – though it is from Romeo who at the time is mooning over someone else – an illusion of love, to be compared with the reality represented by Juliet! The ancient family grudge in which the lovers are reluctantly embroiled is made clear. Our sympathies are engaged. The play (as Dawson points out) starts with a noisy and sudden incident, illustrating the family feud in which the lovers are caught up (Dawson, 1970, p. 34). This has to be established first, and to enable us to see the domestic impact, the play begins 'below stairs' with servants. As it unravels we see that all the characters are 'fortune's fools', the element of chance is strong, and yet there is also a terrible inevitability. Every positive element is countered by its opposite, and this is emphasized by events and the language itself. Weddings are juxtaposed with funerals, day with night, bawdy comedy with romantic love.

In the second act it would seem that the forces of life are winning and the secret marriage of the lovers takes place. But Romeo is sent a challenge. In the third act Romeo kills the challenger and jeopardizes the fate of the lovers. In the fourth act Juliet seeks to re-establish the forces of good, and is helped by Friar Lawrence to execute a plan of feigned death. In the final act, the forces of death and separation win as Romeo and Juliet die. But their families are (belatedly) reconciled. This is a two-faced ending which demands further consideration. The play seems to wrestle with questions of fate and destiny and whether by human intervention we can divert this threat. (And this is demonstrably a theme in many of Shakespeare's plays.) Here, we are asked to pity the lovers but also to ponder the reasons for the reconciliation with which the play ends, to consider the springs of love (heaven) and the senselessness, damage and self-destructiveness of hate (hell), and to recognize that the sacrifice of love can wipe out 'the ancient grudge' (even though there is no paradise on earth at the end) – that mutual forgiveness is essential. And through all, love shines out. For some then, this play is a domestic tragedy, but for some it is an allegory (a symbolic story) about love (see Vyvyan, 1968).

This is the play, then, which provided the inspiration for Tschaikovsky's music. Here, we have meaning without words or pictures and can study an artist communicating through sound alone.

Tschaikovsky's *Fantasia-Overture, Romeo and Juliet*

There is of course a long tradition of relationships between music and the theatre. Music not only serves drama in quite menial ways as incidental music, but plays an equal part with drama in opera. Many composers have taken their inspiration from the theatre. Overtures are a particular musical category and they are of two sorts, those that refer thematically to what is to follow and those that do not. The artistic requirements of an overture are exacting. It must speak decisively and be appealing, have dignity and importance, grip the audience's attention and prepare it for what follows – and all in a small space. At the age of twenty-eight, Tschaikovsky's mastery of orchestral effect is considered to have been complete, and his own style was fully formed. Although his work is less profound and less subtle in feeling than the great masters, it has spontaneity, humanity, and enormous technical skill. Tschaikovsky's *Fantasia* is a kind of symphonic poem (a term created by Lizst). It does not follow the action of the play in detail. Its aim is 'to produce musically the emotional impact of the drama as a whole rather than to illustrate it scene by scene' (Jacob, 1951, p. 12). The work is constructed firmly on the lines of a symphonic first movement. Like Shakespeare's play, it is a piece of great contrasts. The first-scene feud between the Montagues and Capulets provides an invitation to invent a powerful fiery 'first subject', while the love of Romeo and Juliet calls for a second subject which is made up of a group of lyrical themes. Further contrasts come from an ecclesiastical theme which refers to Friar Lawrence and the secret marriage. The work 'glows with the enthusiasm and stormy impetuosity of youth mingled with rich romanticism' (Jacob, 1951, p. 12).

These two examples then (together with *West Side Story* which remakes the story in modern terms) enable us to explore some ideas of what is inherent in our response to drama and music. These are: the notion of performance and script; stage and frame; action and tension, improvisation and composition. Much of the following is shaped by what I learned as a student from Sam Dawson and to Dawson (1970).

Responding to music and drama

Performance and script

Plays and music are, normally, scripted. But it is in performance, not on paper, that they find their proper fulfilment. The primacy of performance is endemic to drama and music. The nature of plays and of music has been and will always be determined by the conditions under which they are able to be acted or played. Professional practice is, to these extents, akin to the performing arts. It is to some extent 'scripted' (and increasingly so because of the fashion for protocols and mandatory 'guidelines'), and yet the script *has* to be left behind in the performance and it is the conditions of the specific 'practice' which determine the kind of performance. It is the performance and not the script that is 'complete', just as a play or score, read rather than performed, is incomplete. But this is not, of course, to use the term 'performance' in a pejorative sense which would suggest that professional practice lacks genuineness.

When we read a play or score we put ourselves (consciously or otherwise) into the position of the producer and company or conductor and orchestra. (And it is here too that professionals –

and managers – might learn from the appreciation of drama and music.) Indeed, as Dawson argues 'any critical discussion of a play that is not in some sense the sketch of a production is not likely to enhance our understanding' (Dawson, 1970, p. 2). He also notes that producers are often forced to answer questions which either do not occur to readers, or which readers are content to leave unanswered, and that 'dramatic literature requires a responsiveness, not just of mind but of the whole body, so that only in performance (solitary though that performance may be) does the whole work realize itself' (Dawson, 1970, p. 3). He concludes that 'the ideal commentator on drama would combine a scrupulous critical concern with the text with as close a concern as possible with the necessities and potentialities of actual performance' (Dawson, 1970, p. 6–7).

Stage and frame, involvement and judgement

The dramatist's first and major task is to seize hold of and retain our attention for several hours (the composer of music does the same if for a somewhat shorter but even more concentrated period) and evoke in us a response to what we are seeing and/or hearing. How he or she involves the audience is therefore also of interest to someone wishing to respond to or appreciate drama (and music). This, then, is about the manner in which the audience is drawn to relate to the play or musical composition – about how the dramatist or composer builds up expectation, creates tension, deploys 'dramatic moments', increases complexity and depth, arouses emotions, or draws us to be judgemental about motive and cause, or tempts us to try to solve the problem ahead of the ending. An appreciation of a play or a piece of music (such as was offered above) will enable a reader to see these things more clearly.

The intention of drama is at one level to induce the audience to believe that what is happening on stage is happening for real – and is happening now! Indeed, the Greeks believed that what happened on stage should be limited to the probabilities and possibilities of real life (and thus that the time and place depicted on stage should be limited so that the natural duration of the performance paralleled the duration of the action in the play). How the play is presented to the audience – how it is 'framed' – is germane here. The picture frame stage which resembles a room with one wall removed, or a garden peered at over an invisible fence, together with 'real-life' language is meant to create the illusion of 'reality', and immediacy. But plays were not always presented in such closely 'framed' stages, and as Dawson points out, the drama of, for example, Shakespeare, comes not from the setting and the physical action on stage, *but from the language of the play*. It is the language which provides the real 'frame' of the play. It is that which 'establishes for the audience what are the criteria of possibility and probability; movement, gesture, properties and scenery are auxiliaries which, ideally speaking, should *grow out* of the creative language' (Dawson, 1970, pp. 8–9).

However, a play is a world within a world, and the audience that loses itself totally in the action, that surrenders its vision entirely to the limited vision of the action on the stage becomes dislocated from any means of judgement. (And here, in professional practitioners' terms, is an argument for reflective practice which ensures that the 'particular' is related to general professional issues.) The setting of the play (the social world the characters inhabit) limits both the range and depth of the action. Somehow we, as audience, also need to be aware of other worlds beyond this, and even perhaps of our own. We must maintain our distance so that we can understand the action in ways that no one inside the play can. We must inhabit several arenas at once. How the dramatist enables us to do this is inevitably of interest. The action and the language must be at once compelling and vivid so that we are involved, and yet there must be language and pauses, gestures and emphases which enable us to disengage from the hurly-burly of action. Professional practitioners developing their practice and an appreciation of it would find useful examples here.

One of the chief means of providing vivid and compelling action in drama is to create moments of tension. A consideration of some of these techniques is also instructive for a practitioner preparing to recognize and write an appreciation of his or her own practice.

Action and tension

The dramatist, then, both 'establishes the limits of the world which the play will inhabit' and 'seizes our attention by creating a situation which is interesting in itself, and which arouses expectation of further situations which may develop out of it' (Dawson, 1970, p. 29). The beginning of Shakespeare's *Romeo and Juliet* illustrates this well, as the summary above shows. We quickly become aware of both short- and long-term expectations about the lovers and the family quarrel. We become curious to see how it all works out – even when we know the end. We are drawn into the action, launched into the middle of it by the first scene where we have a sense of eavesdropping on family matters. Dawson points out that 'tension' is a word bound to occur in any discussion of drama. He adds – significantly for critics and for practitioners interested in critical appreciation:

> All works of art are fully grasped through the perception of the interrelatedness of their parts, and in drama the relation between parts is characteristically one of tension. (Dawson, 1970, p. 30)

He adds that there are many forms and sources of tension in drama. He gives as an instance of these the different ways in which a speech is understood, either between two characters or between audience and character. The audience in *Romeo and Juliet*, for example, hear 'Fate' and 'Destiny' evoked often by the characters but know in advance, as those on stage do not, of the impending tragedy. Tension is also evident between ideas and is often high-lighted by the imagery of a play. (Again we have already seen this in the imagery of *Romeo and Juliet* – see the summary above.) Dawson also says: 'a play remains in a state of imperfect equilibrium until the completion of the action, and the most simple and striking example of this tension is suspense' (Dawson, 1970, p. 30). He later adds that surprise – 'a sudden introduction of a new element into an established situation so as to immediately trans-form it' (Dawson, 1970, p. 32) – is another example of tension. And he makes the point that in respect of both suspense and sur-prise there is usually a subtle element introduced because 'we know, in fact, when we are watching a cliff-hanger, that the hero and heroine will survive' (Dawson, 1970, p. 32). However, he also makes the point that Shakespeare rarely if ever uses pure and unsubtle suspense or surprise, and that the audience has in fact been prepared for all the strikingly dramatic moments in the plays (and this is clearly true of Romeo and Juliet). Of all this he then says:

> This is the supreme art of the dramatist, the creation of an underly-ing sense of what the action must be, which does not emerge into full consciousness until the action is at last completed, so that there

is a perpetual tension between this, and what is happening at any particular moment. The conclusion of the play, an analogy with music being most appropriate here, is like the final major chord of a symphony which has throughout been there *in potentia*, which we never actually hear until the end, and which sets the seal on our intuitive understanding of what has gone before. (Dawson, 1970, pp. 33–34)

Such a sense of audience would stand professionals who write about their practice in good stead, as we shall see in Part Three of this book.

So far we have considered music and drama in their traditional forms, as scripted prior to performance. But this was not, of course, how Shakespeare originally worked. Where a play or a musical composition contains elements which are not scripted, or where they are totally improvised (as indeed, much if not all professional practice is), then other characteristics of the performing arts emerge, and some of these are vitally important in helping practitioners to understand their own work. This includes the importance of cooperation and teamwork where intent listening to others as well as playing one's own part is a basic requirement.

Improvisation

Schön has long since made the point that there is always improvisation in skilled performance – even when it is scripted. He points to the need for *variations* in performance, noting that a skilled performer 'adjusts his responses to variations in phenomena. In his moment-by-moment appreciations of a process, he deploys a wide-ranging repertoire of [previous] images of contexts and actions' (Schön, 1987a, p. 29). He cites a cellist who stood in at the last minute in an orchestra playing a piece hitherto entirely unknown, who sight-read the score, sensing 'at each moment the direction of its development, picking up in his own performance the lines of development already laid down by others . . . [his] interpretation guided by his emerging sense of the whole' (Schön, 1987a, p. 30).

He has also cited conversation (collective verbal improvisation) and jazz as examples of improvisation without a script. He notes that in both cases participants listen to each other and themselves as they feel where the music (or conversation) is going and adjust their part accordingly. He says:

a figure announced by one performer will be taken up by another, elaborated, turned into a new melody. Each player makes on-line inventions and responds to surprises triggered by the inventions of the other players. But the collective process of musical invention is organized around an underlying structure. There is a common schema of meter, melody, and harmonic development that gives the piece a predictable order. In addition, each player has at the ready a repertoire of musical figures around which he can weave variations as the opportunity arises. (Schön, 1987a, p. 30)

He then makes the point that improvisation 'consists in varying, combining, and recombining a set of figures within a schema that gives coherence to the whole piece' (Schön, 1987a, p. 30). He refers to this as reflecting-in-action on the music they are collectively making. In conversation, too, some elements are predictable and some are not; 'participants pick up and develop themes of talk, spinning out variations on their repertoire of things to say' (Schön, 1987a, p. 30). He notes that:

at times it falls into conventional routines – the anecdote with side comments and reactions, for example, or the debate – which develop according to a pace and rhythm of interaction that the participants seem, without conscious deliberation, to work out in common within the framework of an evolving division of labor. At other times, there may be surprises, unexpected turns of phrase or directions of development to which participants invent on-the-spot responses. (Schön, 1987a, pp. 30–31)

This example is echoed by Sloboda (1985), in a digression from his discussion of musical improvisation (see below), when he discusses improvisation in relation to his own work in seminars. He says that when he began to lecture professionally he was terrified of the question session that followed his set-piece. He describes it thus:

I was afraid of many things: not knowing the answer to a question, having some devastating criticism pointed at my work, not being able to put together a fluent reply without preparation. These fears began to subside as (a) I realized that I had a natural advantage over my audience; that of knowing the details of my own material, through many months of involvement with it, far better than anyone in the audience, and (b) I developed a repertoire of ways of handling awkward or unpleasant questions without faltering or becoming confused. The most important thing in situations like this is not to provide the *best* answer, but to provide *an* answer of some respectability with the fluency and immediacy that signals competence. (Sloboda, 1985, p. 148)

He also makes the point that every act of story-telling that is not verbatim recall is an act of improvisation. Thus we can see that there are available more examples of improvisation from which to learn than we sometimes recognize. But of course it is in music that they find their apotheosis.

Improvisation and composition

In his book on the cognitive psychology of music, Sloboda raises an interesting question about the composer as improviser. He notes that in an improvised *performance* (perhaps of a jazz musician, jazz being a Western form of music in which improvisation is paramount), the first idea that the musician has must work first time. But he also notes that a composer is an improviser, citing Beethoven: 'the same man who could chisel away at a theme for 20 years could also produce live compositions of extreme accomplishment' (Sloboda, 1985, p. 139).

He then attempts to distinguish between composition and improvisation. The improviser does not have to be continually referring back, he says, to the detailed working out of earlier sections, as it may be argued a composer must (and as exemplified in Tschiakovsky's *Romeo and Juliet* overture, with its pre-figuring and recapitulating of the key themes). He can 'rely on the given constraints of the [musical] form together with his own "style" to give musical unity' (Sloboda, 1985, p. 139). The improviser is not a long term planner. He or she has a relatively rigid formal frame within which to improvise, which dictates the overall structure of the performance and shapes all improvisations within the piece. Sloboda likens this to the frames of reference in story-telling (where the key elements are 'given' but different tellers can embellish the details as they please, and where the terms 'theme', 'variation' and 'fugue' are familiar). He adds that such structures allow both listeners and the teller to keep track of the complex internal details of a composition. He says:

> in music, we may equate [these] 'frames' with characteristic harmonic or melodic progressions that underlie many different types of music. For instance, cadences are harmonic frames; particular types of melodic movement, such as scales, arpeggios, gap-fill or changing

note patterns ... are melodic frames. As in stories, many of these frames can be filled quite simply, with a couple of notes or chords, but can be fleshed out with various types of embellishment. (Sloboda, 1985, p. 140)

He adds later that 'when such structures are known by listeners they are able to appreciate the function of present events', and, anticipating future constraints, they can appreciate the art that produces relevant innovations exactly as required. He instances the 'chorus' and solo 'break' in jazz, where an individual performer comes to the fore in an innovatory fashion for a fixed number of bars before leading back into the next chorus. He says: 'a listener who knows this structure can realize that the solo is about to end, and wonder how on earth the soloist is going to return satisfactorily from his harmonic and melodic excursions . . . . When such a performer does 'get home', in an appropriate but novel way, the listener can derive satisfaction, of a kind unavailable to someone ignorant of the structures.

The twelve bar blues and the thirty-two bar song are the two primary jazz forms. The melody is often a 'standard' song, which at first is played straightforwardly. The repeated improvisations retain the basic harmonic sequence. The essence of the improvisation being in the melodic line. What gives jazz its special character is the types of melody, rhythms and harmony which are the basic building blocks for larger sequences. But jazz improvisation is not learnt by being armed with a list of characteristic chords and progressions. It is learned 'through listening intently to other musicians and performing with them. Books and notation are not necessary'. Indeed, many great jazz players do not read music (see Sloboda, 1985, p. 143).

The jazz performer can build up a repertoire of things that have worked well in the past. The jazz improviser enjoys improvisation because there will always be something he can play (Sloboda, 1985, p. 149). Very often, too, wrong notes can be used positively, and the improviser is relaxed, knowing that, wherever he lands up there are 'a dozen different ways of getting from there to the next place'. This confidence, which he argues is the hallmark of impromptu accomplishment, comes from the 'availability of plenty of escape routes' (Sloboda, 1985, p. 148). Much of this will have echoes for the professional practitioner.

He notes that there is often less real improvisation on a concert platform – improvisatory devices which have worked well in the past, or even rehearsed improvisations being used – because musicians take fewer risks there than they might in 'late-night backroom informal sessions where, amidst a dedicated and sympathetic audience, experiments that fail, as well as those that reach new heights, may be observed' (Sloboda, 1985, p. 149). By comparison, the composer:

> rejects possible solutions until he finds one which seems to be the best for his purposes. The improviser must accept the first solution that comes to hand. In both cases the originator must have a repertoire of patterns and things to do with them that he can call up at will; but in the case of improvisation the crucial factor is the speed at which the stream of invention can be sustained, and the availability of things to do which do not overtax the available resources. In composition, fluency becomes less important; but it is much more important to keep long-term structural goals in sight, and to unify present material with what has gone before. (Sloboda, 1985, p. 149)

Interestingly, he illustrates a simple theme and variation form found in classical, folk and jazz idioms (a typical four phrase theme, of eight bars in length with a pattern AABA (where the second and fourth phrases are repeats of the first phrase and the third phrase is different but stylistically and thematically related) and the following variations repeating the pattern with embellishment and decoration $A^1A^1B^1A^1$; $A^2A^2B^2A^2$, etc). He then cites (oral) story-telling as a known set of episodes which make up a set plot but whose detailed characteristics of setting, speech and colour are elaborated and embellished to keep the plot fresh. Those elaborations, he points out, must be appropriately selected, or omitted on the basis of the hearer's knowledge and expectations. Performers and listeners within a culture will know about stereotypical ways of filling in such details. The composer and improviser achieve aesthetic impact by finding novel or surprising ways of embellishing the story (frame) without changing its basic character.

The above is an attempt to provide some of the language for responding to the Arts, which professional practitioners may find helpful in recognizing and useful in responding to the artistic elements of their own practice. From this it is now possible to define rather more clearly what is meant by the word 'appreciation'.

Responding to artistry: key definitions in critical appreciation

This second section of the chapter offers some definitions of terms relating to critical appreciation as an activity. These are: analysis, interpretation and appreciation. It also looks in some detail at the role of critic as connoisseur.

Critical appreciation: a further clarification

Critical appreciation involves both a critical response to a piece of art and a shaping of that response into a commentary. These processes harness both critical analysis and critical interpretation. A clarification of these processes, as they relate to responding to the Arts, will now be attempted. A clarification of the role of connoisseur and critic will also be offered, drawing on the work of Eisner. It will be assumed here that the reader will, in reading this section, bear in mind the foregoing sections of this chapter and the previous chapter, thus having readily available some practical examples of art and of the language of appreciation in the Arts.

Analysis

Analysis is a process in which the components of an activity or an object are separated out into categories for consideration. Analysis claims to be an objective and neutral activity. But its apparent objectivity hides a number of value judgements that have to be made in order to categorize in the first place, and a number of assumptions, including the idea that the whole is always a simple sum of the parts. Put another way, an interesting question to ask about analysis is how far it allows one to respond, or prevents one from responding, holistically to the whole object or process. In contrast to the idea that analysis is an appropriate response to art is the view that a critic needs to begin in humility the task of offering an intelligent and challenging but appreciative critique, needs to start with a sense of wonder that something has been created out of nothing, and consequently ought to hold at bay the kind of arrogance so easily associated with the (apparent) omniscience of being able to dissect a work of art. But the fact remains that analysis must play its part in providing background information to inform a response to art. At best it pays the artist the compliment of ensuring that the detail of his or her work is recognized.

Interpretation

Interpretation, by contrast, is a process which offers a view or views of the nature and meaning of an activity or an object. Such a process proceeds from considering an *overall* view of the activity or object. It is admittedly subjective, and takes account of its subjectivity in its presentation of its view(s). Essentially it is not about breaking the activity or object down into components but about viewing it in an overall way – in order to see it better, to explain it, or to try to say something about what it might mean, what it has to say or what can be said about it. An example in literary criticism is what used to be called the bio-critical approach. The intention here was to convey a sense of the writer's achievement set against the background of his time. It conveyed an overall impression, referring to an appraisal of individual works used to illustrate the generalizations made about the writer. But, of course, the personality of the 'interpreter' is also important here. As Daiches said:

> The success of this kind of criticism depends on its author's ability to handle the various elements of which it is composed in such a way to build up a tone, an atmosphere, which reflects in some way the special qualities of the writer who is being criticised. But the tone is never wholly subdued to its subject: there is always the critic's personality before us, with the critic's preferences and prejudices, his references to pet authors ... and favourite controversies ...
> (Daiches, 1963, p. 286)

By contrast to both analysis and interpretation, critical appreciation starts with trying to recognize and understand what the artist is offering.

Critical appreciation

Essentially, art results from the artist seeing anew and then sharing his or her version of that vision. Critical appreciation, then, is a process in which the artist's vision (both that which the artist was conscious of, and that which the critic sees even when the artist may not have been overtly aware of it) is recognized holistically and responded to – critically and analytically. The critic here seeks to understand the artist's vision and to get to know the artist better (for the sake of responding to the art).

Appreciation is justified by detailed reference to the piece of art, and to its history and the tradition within which or in opposition to which it was fashioned. This process seeks to consider the artistic activity or object from many points of view, balancing appreciative response with close analytical description, seeking to set it in a context that helps to make sense of it, seeing in it meanings beyond the surface and seeing it as representative of something beyond itself.

A critical appreciation, presented as a commentary, seeks to convey a sense of the artist's achievement set against the background of his or her time and informed by some knowledge about the artist. Thus the context of the work comes under scrutiny. (Its historical setting and the traditions within which that work has been created are significant in helping us to understand it.) And in addition to all that, the personal qualities, knowledge and understanding, history and traditions, values and beliefs of the critic (or 'appreciator') are also important, inevitably come through and need to be acknowledged.

It will be apparent from this that the role of judge, in terms of the merit of a piece of art, comes *behind* the task of recognition and response. Armstrong, by reference to considering the value of paintings, helps us here by saying:

> appropriate reasons for judging artistic value concern the exploitation of the ... art-form, the manner in which content has been formed, the importance of the content as formed. And such reasons have to be concerned with the works as intrinsically valuable and as irreplaceable objects of attention. Such reason-giving traces an individual's appreciation of a particular work. But to be relevant to appreciation, the reasons have to be couched in an a-personal way. That is, such reasons are cast without reference to the fact that it is I who am looking at the painting. (Armstrong, 1996, p. 154)

He adds later:

> if a work sustains the judgement that it is of high artistic merit, and on similar grounds, across a wide range of judges, then this gives ground for thinking that the judgement is inter-subjectively valid, and that those who disagree with it have flawed judgement with respect to that work. (Armstrong, 1996, p. 156)

The above clarifications have to some extent been necessary because, as in all things, fashion has affected views about what is appropriate under the heading of 'criticism'. The following gives a brief illustration of this by reference to literary criticism in the later twentieth century. As will be quickly apparent from this, all these fashions have some important things to say about criticism. (For a detailed exploration of the following, see Bennett and Royle, 1995, pp. 10–18.)

Fashions in literary criticism

In the post-war period the major fashion for literary criticism was that known as the 'new criticism' which established the principles of 'practical criticism'. This involved responding to literature in respect of its form – the words on the page – rather than factors such as the 'life of the author and his or her intentions or the historical and ideological context in which the text was produced' (Bennett and Royle, 1995, p. 11). Although the 'new critics' considered such matters interesting, they did not see them as central to a consideration of the text itself, which they saw as self-sufficient – as aesthetic objects made of words. They argued that to try to take account of the background of the author and also the reactions and responses of readers was to introduce alien and extraneous factors. The words of the text were what must be given scrupulous attention. They were objective, whereas the reader's response was subjective. This movement created its own canon of literary works and authors.

By the late 1960s and increasingly in the 1970s and 1980s, an approach known as 'reader–response criticism' gained ground. For this group of theorists, including Stanley Fish (a leading American proponent of this approach), an intelligent reading of the text could not exclude the role of the reader. Indeed, the meaning of the text is created through reading and relies on the work of the reader. They therefore attempt to plot the process of reading and the role of the reader. They also make way for the acceptability of far more interpretations. However, this is, as Bennett and Royle point out (Bennett and Royle, 1995, p. 12), a Pandora's box, opening the way to personal and highly subjective (and often rather immature) criticism (because the idiosyncratic concerns brought to the text were seen as of more significance than the text). As a way of escaping this problem, Stanley Fish has argued that any individual reader is part of a community and that an individual's criticism should also relate to the views of the critical community (rather in the way that Armstrong does above).

During the 1980s and 1990s the political dimensions of reading have become increasingly central to critical debate. Literary texts have been read in terms of power relations, and this has included increased attention to questions of gender and race. Questions have been raised about how different 'reading as a woman' is from 'reading as a man', and about colonization, ethnic difference, racial oppression and discrimination.

Finally, a poststructuralist or deconstructive approach to criticism has become fashionable in the 1990s and has been seen as part of the *fin de siècle* attitude of boredom with and destruction of scholarly 'enlightenment'. Poststructuralists are unsure whether the reader or the text comes first. Is the role of the reader determined by the text, or is the text determined by the role of the reader? Deconstructive theories of reading argue that both models are valuable, and explore the space between these two possibilities, seeking to highlight how every reading and every text is unpredictable. Deconstruction is interested in ways in which the text demands a 'faithful' reading *and* an individual response. It emphasizes the unsettling experience of reading.

Thus it is clear that the term 'criticism' in reference to the appreciation of the Arts (and in this case, of literature in particular) can involve some differences of emphasis. But these differences only serve to emphasize the overall similarities, which are the characteristics we have already offered as a definition. The work of Eisner will now help us to begin to set all this in a more professional context.

Connoisseurship and criticism

In *The Art of Educational Evaluation* (published in America in the face of and in opposition to the scientific approach to education so familiar in Britain today) Eisner pressed the importance of intimation, metaphor, analogy, poetic insight and the shift to autobiographical form (Eisner, 1985, p. 90) as being one of the best ways of capturing the quality of experience in good professional practice. (He referred specifically to teaching, but the comments apply equally to all the caring professions.) He cited 'the cultivation of productive idiosyncrasy' as one of the prime consequences of work in the Arts (Eisner, 1985, p. 91) – and by implication in professional practice. He also considered the role of theory in the cultivation of artistry and concluded that it is diagnostic rather than prescriptive. It provides, he argued, 'a window through which intelligence can look out into the world' (Eisner, 1985, p. 92). Perhaps most importantly, here, Eisner proposed two notions which he argued are useful for considering artistry in teaching. These are educational connoisseurship and educational criticism (see his Chapter 5). He argued that together they can 'contribute to a heightened awareness of the qualities' of professional practice so that professionals 'can become more intelligent within it' (Eisner, 1985, p. 92). In characterizing them he inevitably uses the term appreciation which he usefully defines as 'an awareness and an understanding of what one has experienced which provides a basis for judgement' and as being quite neutral about 'liking' the object of such attention.

He wrote that *connoisseurship* is the art of appreciation (which is private) but what he called *criticism* is more useful for our purposes. Criticism, he said, 'is the art of disclosure (which is public) in that it renders the qualities of the piece of art vivid'. He was at pains to define it as far from dilettante, and in art as doing more than awakening sensibility, rather as demonstrating the history, social context and tradition of the Arts and how they depart from the conventional. This requires an understanding of the various forms that the Arts have taken in the past and understanding the intentions and leading conceptions underlying them. This too seems a useful reminder of what has to be involved in a thorough and systematic piece of practitioner research.

Educational *criticism* , Eisner argued, aims at providing a rendering in linguistic terms of just what it is that the critic has encountered – what it is that is going on in that setting (the qualities that constitute the work, its significance, and the quality of the experience when he or she interacts with it) so that others not possessing that level of connoisseurship can also enter into the work. This is an art in itself, particularly in respect of the way language and form are used. (*This,* I am also arguing, is what practitioner researchers need to develop much more consciously and with an appreciation of the traditions and discipline of criticism itself.) Such criticism draws upon an understanding of the values, history and traditions that lie behind what is happening. It is about perceiving in addition to the superficial and apparent, the covert and the subtle. It is about recognizing what has been rejected as well as what has been accepted. And it is about relating what is seen to the broad practice of which it is part, so that the criteria employed in describing and criticizing are appropriate to it. It is, thus, bent towards re-educating perception. It equips us with new ways of seeing.

> What the critic strives for is to articulate or render those ineffable qualities constituting art in a language that makes them vivid ... the task of the critic is to adumbrate, suggest, imply, connote, render, rather than to attempt to translate. In this task, metaphor and analogy, suggestion and implication are major tools. (Eisner, 1985, p. 92)

This in turn shows the extent to which critical appreciation is itself an art. It reminds us what a long tradition and worthy pedigree it can demonstrate, encompassing as it does writers with interests in philosophical enquiry and critical scholarship (going back to Plato, Aristotle, Horace and Sidney) and practical criticism (including the work of Jonson, Dryden, Dr Johnson, Coleridge and Eliot).

Conclusion

From this, then, I conclude that understanding the concerns and procedures of the artist and of the art critic are not too difficult to explain, grasp or undertake. Further, they have the potential to extend the repertoire of those attempting to see and respond to the artistry of professional practice. And it would seem that they might also be useful for considering the work of practitioners and for enabling practitioner researchers to write about their art, as well as for providing resources for those involved in producing a critical appreciation of the practitioner's practice or writing. Equipped with these ideas, then, let us turn to the practical implications of this work.

Part Three

Cultivating an appreciative eye: some practical processes for professional development and research

8

Appreciation and the development of discernment: recognizing and preparing to capture the artistry in our practice

Introduction to Part Three

This part of the book focuses on practical issues in order to support professionals wishing to investigate the artistry of their practice from within the artistic paradigm and who through this seek new understanding in order to improve their service to patients, clients and pupils or students. The term practitioner researcher is used in this chapter to mean any practitioner or student practitioner who seeks to improve practice in these ways, and where personal practice is the main focus.

The origins of this work are humble but the implications can be far reaching. In starting with a small but well chosen piece of his or her own practice a professional can quickly unravel some of the issues at its core and come to see them as relating to the heart of the profession's practice. Further, by sharing these in public, professionals could ultimately reshape the public's perceptions of practice. As we argued in Fish and Coles (1998), practitioners can be changed by such study, since it increases awareness of the bases of professional actions, decisions, judgements. Primarily it enables professionals to see their practice anew, to recognize and articulate its complexities and the contestable notions and values that lie at its heart, and thus to learn to refine those things which can be developed and live with those which cannot. Appreciating the artistry of professional work can profoundly alter practitioners' understanding of practice and theory, and can equip them to be articulate about this, to think critically about it, to establish different priorities as the basis for practice, and thus effect far-reaching and well-founded changes to practice. It might even lead practitioners to challenge the notion of *evidence*-based practice and work towards the establishment of praxis (*morally*-based practice), and thus reinstate professionalism on a proper foundation. Thus, the understandings that arise from small-scale study can extend and provoke further debate, reshape public understanding and make an impact upon the practitioner in profound ways (see Fish and Coles, 1998, pp. 303–307).

Conducting such a study of one's own work involves investigating the iceberg of one's practice, that is, revealing the depth of thought and feeling beneath our actions (that which is ineffable, unspoken, unacknowledged during practice) and articulating it (perhaps in figurative language) so that it can be learnt from and worked upon. It is demanding work. But colleagues with whom I have explored these matters in practice have found the process liberating, exciting and helpful at a number of levels. Indeed, as editors of the work of one group, Colin Coles and I argued that 'we know of no other activity in professional practice – apart from the rewards of practice itself – which at the same time fulfils the demands for accountability, research, and professional development and provides refreshment of mind and spirit' (Fish and Coles, 1998, p. 59).

The nature of practical research in the artistic/holistic paradigm

As demonstrated in Chapter 5, empirical work in the artistic/holistic paradigm is small scale. The intention here is not to amass large amounts of data but to collect only that information which enables the practitioner researcher to work in detail on understanding a selected piece of practice. One way of operating, which the following chapters support, is to work towards two outcomes: an artistic portrait of a piece of practice, and a critical commentary on the portrait and its production, and on the professional practice which was its subject. It will be necessary to collect and create whatever information is needed to support and enrich the ultimate production of these two central processes in order to do justice to the practice (both its surface and its underlying qualities – theories, values, professional judgements, emotions, improvisations, intuitions). The portrait and the commentary might be thought of as offering two perspectives on practice, and both will be shaped by critical consideration of theory (formal, espoused and theory-in-use), as well as practice.

It should be noted that the portrait of practice is not the same as the usual straightforward narrative or reports of a critical incident, but is an artistic presentation (or interpretation) of a subject which has been deliberately and deliberatively selected and observed, isolated and accentuated, in order to uncover and reveal some deeper truths about that practice, practice in general, and the artistry of practice. This is most likely to be best achieved by embarking on a number of draft sketches of the subject and of matters which provide a context for the subject, from a range of perspectives. When working with a group of health care professionals in exploring these ideas in practice it emerged strongly that investigating practice in this way does involve considerable re-working. (Indeed, we discovered that such re-working needed particular support from us in respect of how to theorize practice and how to harness artistry of expression (see Fish and Coles, 1998).) This process was also helped by working with a colleague or colleagues in a relationship known as 'critical friendship'. This consists of using the services of a colleague to act as a thoughtful (critical) audience to help check out and expand one's ideas and act as a sounding board for the theorizing of one's practice as well as its presentation and communication in writing. This is because understanding practice in order to present a portrait and a commentary involves the need to argue with ourselves and deliberate (with others) – to engage in practical reasoning – about the dilemmas, the inevitably contestable issues that are endemic to professional practice. 'It involves improving practice through systematic critical enquiry where the term critical implies review leading to better understanding of practice and offering potential emancipation from existing traditions or established patterns of practice' (Golby and Appleby, 1995, p. 150).

For the purpose of exploring ideas and preserving draft sketches (as a means of charting the progress of ideas and understanding), an 'artist's notebook' or 'sketchbook' approach is advisable. This is not quite the same as the traditional field diaries of the social sciences paradigms which record chronologically the researcher's investigative activities and ideas. Rather, it is like an artist's workbook and enables the researcher to make preliminary sketches of the projected subject or similar subjects and of a range of contextual ideas and may uncover the need for more observation and investigation before the final portrait is attempted. The portrait itself may *then* be better worked on without interruption for the purpose of seeking further data, since it will be attempting to capture a holistic view of a subject which will be designed to make a holistic impact. Even though the practitioner researcher may be attempting to become more fully an artist in order to improve the artistry of his or her practice, such work, of course, cannot reasonably be judged on its artistic merit since the intention here is professional rather than artistic. For this reason, the critical commentary will (amongst other things) provide the opportunity to indicate how far the portrait has been successful in exploring and revealing the artistry of practice.

With all this in mind, this part of the book is organized as follows. This chapter looks in detail at how to recognize, isolate and begin to set about capturing artistry in professional practice, while Chapter 9 considers ways of creating *draft* portraits of professional practice and the importance in these of seeing the artistry and the practice in its full context – looking at how it relates to the history and traditions of the profession involved, and establishing the situational context. (Reference is made in both chapters to the procedures of critical appreciation as discussed in Part Two.) Ways of refining and shaping this work for its final presentation are the focus of Chapter 10, which draws upon the information about narrative and autobiographical form first discussed in Chapter 6. In the final chapter of this section some principles are considered which can guide the production of a critical commentary upon the portrait of practice and ultimately upon practice itself.

Readers are reminded that producing a sensitive and artistic portrait of practice and a critical commentary of it are creative acts in themselves, so, only the broad principles can be offered here. (Examples across a range of health care professions can be found in Fish and Coles, 1998; examples specific to nursing can be found in Chinn and Watson, 1994; examples specific to teaching can be found in *Educational Theory*, 1995 (volume 45, number 1), which is dedicated to exploring ways in which the Arts can enhance understanding of schools and their curriculum.) What follows, therefore, is designed to offer clarification, advice and some frameworks that will support professionals in attempting to work in this way.

Introduction to this chapter

Where value in the scientific paradigm is founded almost exclusively on quantity, and in the social science paradigms is founded on the moral worth of individuals (their behaviour and their social interactions), in an artistic research paradigm what is valued is a process and/or a piece of professional artistry, and/or a portrait of the artistry of practice and the deeper truths to which these can give us access. (Such professional artistry will, of course, by definition, include a moral dimension.) In order, therefore, to support colleagues' investigations (which will begin with the recognition of and the homing in upon practice and isolating a particular subject in order to consider it critically), this chapter concerns itself with two main issues. The first looks further at what constitutes professional artistry and at what is involved in the processes of its appreciation. The second considers the role in this of case study research.

Professional artistry and its appreciation

There are two key elements to the appreciation of art, which are closely interrelated, but which are here discussed separately for the sake of clarity. One key element is focused upon practice itself (which we have argued is endemically artistic), and might be referred to as *cultivating the discerning eye*. This involves learning to recognize the value – even the holistic quality – of professional practice *and* recognizing its endemic artistry. It is about developing the ability to be open to the overall impact of, and to notice the significant details of, any pieces or processes of professional practice. This involves being willing to focus upon a variety of examples of practice, being prepared to allow them to make their overall impact, and being willing to consider them in detail. It also involves continually working at refining one's understanding of what one is looking at and gradually isolating that which one will consider in even greater detail. By contrast, it does *not* involve having (or even trying to develop) a pre-formed list of elements to look for. Learning to recognize the artistry in practice can however be helped by developing some sense of what distinguishes art from craft on the one hand and routine practice on the other. It is also aided by considering *in principle* what might be recognized as characteristic of that practice which earns the term 'artistic merit', and what would immediately exclude practice from such an accolade.

The other (closely related) key element is focused upon appreciation itself and is about *developing an appreciative cast of mind*. This involves learning to work within the traditions of the critical appreciation of the Arts (having knowledge of, and being able to access information about the ideas and traditions, the expectations and assumptions, the conventional and the original, in critical appreciation, and being conscious of its methods and means) as well as learning to respond through them to professional practice as an art.

Both cultivating a discerning eye and developing an appreciative cast of mind are essentially practical processes and are best learnt in practice. They depend upon being able to access some knowledge about the Arts (of the kind illustrated in Part Two), and are helped by studying examples of writings which have explored the artistry of professional practice – as offered in Chapters 2 and 3 of this book, in Fish and Coles (1998) and in Chinn and Watson (1994). But above all they are achieved by action. What follows is an attempt to clarify some matters about how to set about such cultivation and development.

Recognizing art and artistry

A painter's sketchbook may contain as many words as pictures. Many of these will capture the struggle with ideas which is an inevitable part of understanding the complexity of practice in visual art and the intellectual and practical problems endemic to working as an artist and a professional. In such a sketchbook painters try out ideas – often from several angles. In attempting to explore the artistry of practice, practitioner researchers will find it useful to adopt this same approach. The following attempts to offer some possible starting points, to fuel some ideas (which will need to be considered critically) and to motivate some action, which should provoke practitioner researchers to begin to use that sketchbook.

Starting points

Artistic quality (in art itself as well as in professional practice) is often first grasped by allowing the piece of art or practice to make its impact, and of reporting what it was that made that impact. This is a far cry from setting out to find – as fast as possible – professional competencies and check them off against a pre-selected list. Instead, it involves focusing on pieces of practice which are likely to offer the opportunity to capture a holistic picture of professional artistry and allowing enough time for them each to make their overall impact, and then (and only then) considering their detail. Just as a painter chooses to sketch some scene which pleases him or her – which attracts the eye – so the professional practitioner should choose a small incident which attracts his or her attention. A useful beginning can be made by starting (much as in an art gallery) with the work of a colleague – work to which one is naturally drawn and which by common consent offers particular examples of considerable artistry – or one's own work with which one has been instinctively pleased. (In one's own work it will be easier to uncover the tacit levels.) Not all will bring instant insight, though some may. In some cases closer scrutiny may result in a reiteration of qualities already known about (but now understood personally), in some cases it may produce disappointment when the impact turns out to be less than was expected or when the detail examined proves it unconvincing as art, or when the end result leads the observer to respect the practice without liking it. As we shall see below, this does not matter as it is possible to appreciate artistic failure as well as success, because it will have provided valuable experience in appreciation. (In the context of the Arts, just as 'criticism' is not necessarily negative, so 'appreciation' is not necessarily positive.)

But, if the discerning eye is to be developed, then responding to congenial pieces of practice which are readily characterizable as artistry needs soon to give way to focusing on pieces which (because their artistry is less obvious or less extensive) make more demands of the appreciative critic. Indeed, a project which might be a highly suitable topic for an insider practitioner researcher is one in which (by focusing upon a number of pieces of personal practice) he or she traced the development of his or her professional artistry (at both a practical and a theoretical level), and considered the work in the context of the work of a range of fellow practitioners and a range of theoretical perspectives. This would reveal the practitioner's progress and growth in artistry, discernment and taste, and could reveal the impact of the resulting understandings upon personal practice. In fact, this approach could be adjusted in scope and depth for use from undergraduate to doctoral level, and from formal research to professional development.

Such work might begin by considering carefully, and then extending further or refuting the following distinctions.

Some important distinctions

Art and craft are closely related, the term 'art' being, in many cases, reserved for something deserving the greater praise because it is original, unique, unrepeatable, whereas craft suggests a predetermined product (which need not have involved artistry), begun with the deliberate intention of repeated and regular production and being therefore of lower intrinsic value than art. Although the word 'art' has undergone many shifts of meaning, as Armstrong points out, it almost always means that something has intrinsic value, has been created with artistry and is irreplaceable (Armstrong, 1996, p. 35). The following five key points can now be made about professional artistry.

Professional artistry, then, is firstly a term only accorded to that professional practice which achieves the profession's moral ends. It may, in addition, achieve lesser functions at the same time – as long as these are not in conflict with the moral ends. We have already established, following Aristotle, that all professional practice potentially has intrinsic value as offering moral good to clients (the good that health practitioners seek being health and perhaps education). (It may be remembered that according to Aristotle, action in which the end product is not an object but is the realization of morally worthwhile good, is termed *praxis*; see, for example, W. Carr, 1995.) Such good cannot be *made* outside the practice and then delivered to it, but can only be done within it. That is, the ends cannot be absolutely designed in advance of engaging in the practice. Although they might be *formulated* in theory, they are not fixed, but are mutable and develop as the practice develops. And they are only intelligible in terms of the traditions of good (health and education) which are being practised. But of course not all such practice achieves the intended good, and some (sadly) settles happily for lesser and more immediate ends – some of which can actually turn out to conflict with the client's ultimate good.

Secondly, if it is to be acknowledged as involving artistry, professional practice must be significantly valuable *as a whole*. The merit (intrinsic value) of such professional artistry depends on its properties being in a particular arrangement which only a consideration of the whole view of that practice will reveal. (If one of the properties which make up that practice is changed, the value of that practice as artistry will be lost.) This is not about what the practice looks like at the level of its visible characteristics, but about how the visible and the invisible characteristics of professional practice come together at the same time in harmony, in such a way that they are particularly appropriate to the moral intention and the content of that practice. The term 'artistry', then, here indicates that the practitioner has used personal resources to achieve his or her profession's moral ends by means of visible and invisible actions and ideas which are in balance with those ends – are in harmony with them, are integrated with them to the point of unity. (This unity often makes it hard to recognize the individual parts involved, and some elements will remain mysterious.)

Further, professional artistry is, then, emphatically more than simply deploying, in a routine way, some well-honed skills in order to achieve some pre-determined short-term professional ends. Well-honed skills may underlie artistic ability (though may not be prerequisites of it), but on their own, such skills do not explain or count as professional artistry. Professional ends determined by those outside the profession may be a requirement of today's practitioner, but the practitioner who works with artistry will couch these in wider moral terms and see them as a personal responsibility. Thus, artist practitioners whose practice is of high quality match the demands of the moral ends they are seeking to achieve to some highly appropriate and well-executed professional skills and capacities and positive personal qualities. And such a match causes them to operate in a style which cannot fully be done justice to by breaking down the component parts of their practice, because there will always be in it some irreducible element of mystery. It can therefore only be referred to as the ability to act with professional artistry. It consists of a *whole process* – some aspects of which are invisible to the eye – in which many things are happening at the same time or in which one set of actions is simultaneously achieving many different ends, but which will never yield fully to analysis. This is why figurative and poetic language which works on several levels at once is best equipped to capture and do justice to it and why neither analysis nor multi-perspective interpretation will unlock the details. It is this which (in terms used in the Arts too) makes professional practice both intrinsically valuable and irreplaceable (original). And it is all this which leads those concerned with artistry to be unable in simple terms to define 'good practice' (unlike those who take a technical rational view and who seek to list individual and predetermined competencies and by this means to exclude all else from consideration).

Thirdly, the term 'professional artistry' is not merited according to the degree of artistic performance exhibited. Clearly, some professional work could contain a strong element of 'good performance' (artistic content) and yet still not have a high value as professional artistry. If, for example, the activity involved is simple and trivial (or the intention is more focused upon demonstrating artistry than on proper professional intentions), however well it is performed it will not be high level artistry. Equally, performance only takes account of that which is visible, and as we pointed out in our iceberg metaphor for practice, nine-tenths of practice is below the surface.

Fourthly, the value of the content of such practice is also germane to whether or not practice involves professional artistry. To count as artistry, a piece of professional practice has to be worth doing in the first place. (This would exclude practice which was primarily motivated by the need to put on a show to an outside observer or inspector.) If professional practice is not of high enough value to be of intrinsic merit and considered irreplaceable, then it is not valuable as professional artistry.

Finally – but significantly – such practice must also exhibit imagination in harnessing capacities and skills to ends such that the practice is more than a 'routine activity, routinely conducted'. To qualify as characterizable as professional artistry, then, practice must be imaginative in responding, *in the practice*, to the practical problems that arise and in selecting and harnessing skills and capacities that are perfectly matched to intention, but which may not have been considered during the preparation stage. (Though this *alone* is not enough for practice to count as art.) Armstrong notes that:

> artistry and imagination are the *abilities* characteristic of the production of works of art, without being the unique determinants of artistic value. The exercise of artistry and imagination is *not sufficient* for the creation of a work of high artistic merit, although the exercise of artistry and imagination is a *necessary* condition for high artistic value. (Armstrong, 1996, p. 53)

The study of artistry is more than an empirical study. There is (as I long since argued) no blueprint for good practice which is truly artistic, though it is possible to have a blueprint for a technical rational version of 'good practice'. (Readers will now be in a position to produce a critique of the list offered at the end of Chapter 3.) Rather, we can only learn from the consideration of examples which we have to seek out in practice and which we can come to recognize as particular examples of what is generalizable as professional artistry. It is for this reason that developing the discerning eye and cultivating an appreciative cast of mind involves time spent in looking at and responding to the impact of a range of practice. Almost any piece of practice which exists as an entity may well exemplify artistry and will provide useful experience in critical appreciation – except those lacking in artistry in ways discussed above.

If this offers some further comments on professional artistry, what then of the second key element mentioned above as necessary for embarking on the study of professional artistry – namely the processes and nature of critical appreciation?

Appreciation

Appreciation – in the context of art and artistry – involves grasping the valuable qualities of something which is seen, responded to and discussed as a whole entity, and taking proper account of its full context (the history and traditions as well as the specific situation out of which it springs). It is – as we have already noted – about being able to let the art make its impact, and being able to report what it was about it that made the impact (about being able to give an explanation of how and why that piece of art, or the artistic performance or process, is valuable, and what it promises and offers its audience). And it is about giving good reasons for (in support of) our evaluations (our judgement of the quality), which discuss those qualities the art itself really does have. What is sometimes called 'criticism' – in the term literary criticism – is about trying to be *self-conscious* about (to recognize and make explicit) our evaluations of literature. This 'self-consciousness' is not about becoming more aware of oneself, but rather should involve forgetting self and our hang-ups, and responding intelligently and creatively to the art involved.

A highly significant, and sometimes neglected element in all this is the context. The situation out of which the practice has sprung needs to be considered from a number of points of view, each one of which can affect the practice deeply, such that in ignoring them our response to and our understanding of that practice might be seriously distorted. The physical context needs to be carefully explored and documented, and often conveys far more than is at first obvious.

For example, much can be deduced in terms of a practitioner's values from the lay-out of the room in which the practice takes place. Where there is choice, the positioning of key pieces of furniture often indicates how the practitioner sees his or her role, and where furniture is fixed, the use to which it is put often indicates how human relationships are perceived. Novelists have long since known this and some even go so far as to indicate character by means of detailed setting. An example being James Joyce's story in *Dubliners* called 'A Painful Case', which opens with a lengthy description (in terms of look, smell, sound and even touch and taste) of the main character's living room (Joyce, 1965 [1914]). But equally important is an understanding of the history and traditions within which a particular piece of professional practice falls. This means the need always to recognize the history of the practitioner and of his or her practice (so that one piece of practice is seen as part of the larger whole of that person's normal work), and consider it in relation to the history and traditions of the profession within which he or she is working.

For example, I have in my possession a video tape made in 1990 of a teacher in Hungary using an experiential approach to teaching a small piece of mathematics to nine-year-olds. To my eyes it seems a crass and fairly unsuccessful attempt to engage children in meaningful activities so that they gain insight from them and discover new relationships and achieve new understandings. This is mainly because the teacher keeps control of everything they do and does much of the thinking for them while they go meticulously through motions she dictates and which she has previously planned. However, given her normal didactic approach, the traditional views at that time of her country on what constitutes 'teaching', and the traditions of the teaching profession in that country, she was actually operating bravely in new and adventurous ways (even though I would have suggested a different approach to beginning to use this method).

This too has its parallels in art appreciation and, indeed, appreciation of any of the Arts. For example, an understanding of the Bruegel painting discussed in Chapter 6, and an appreciation of its value as art depends essentially on recognizing when, within the history of visual art, and within what artistic traditions Bruegel was painting. What we can expect from the painting and what he can achieve as an artist are shaped by these matters. Langford makes these points. He refers to Gombrich, the great art historian, who 'points out that we cannot understand the history of art – why indeed, art *has* a history – without recognizing the fact that painters paint as they do primarily because they have learnt to do so from their predecessors' (Langford, 1985, p. 3). He adds later:

> limits are set to the scope for innovation on the part of even the greatest painters by the tradition to which they belong . . . . What a tradition gives to a painter, in addition to and even more important than skills and techniques, is a way of seeing the world [and therefore ways of doing too] . . . . To introduce a new style – in other words a new way of seeing – is not [easy], and it is the work of those who have managed to do so which provides the landmarks in the history of art. (Langford, 1985, pp. 7–8)

He says later that a 'way of seeing which a tradition provides' can be modified by both external influences (the discovery of traditions from another country) and 'through the personal vision and creative activity of its most outstanding practitioners'. He adds:

> The history of art is in fact the history of such modifications. Creative individuality of one sort or another is made possible by the relevant tradition rather than being ruled out by it . . . [though] traditions differ greatly in the scope which they provide for individual expression. (Langford, 1985, p. 21)

Appreciating artistry and our own professional practice, then, involves being able to respond to the overall impact of an artefact or artistic process – seen within its context – and depends upon being able to explain to ourselves what is valuable about it. Such an explanation is couched in terms of the valuable (or undesirable) qualities of the object or process as a whole. And this in turn is about what one brings to the object or process in the first place, in terms of knowledge and experience, sensitivity, imagination and values. It involves a *cultivated* response to the impact of the whole and an ability to point to features within it (which *are there* for everyone to discover) (see Armstrong, 1996, pp. 16–19).

Appreciation is about valuing something artistic for appropriate reasons (reasons which are appropriate to the traditions of that kind of art and appropriate to the critical response to such art). Such appreciation must be expressed in terms of the qualities which the object or process appreciated really does have. However, it is not *necessary* to like as well as to appreciate a piece of art. It is possible to recognize that others find in it something valuable and to understand and even agree with the reasons for this, without actually enjoying or liking it. (One 'does not have to be stranded at the end of someone else's judgement'.) Equally (on the other hand), the justification of the judgement of quality is independent of *who* happens to provide it (see Armstrong, 1996, p. 22).

To be acceptable *as* appreciation, the reasons given for something having artistic merit must demonstrably apply to the work in question, and be appropriate to the establishing of such merit. They must be real reasons for valuing (rather than liking or enjoying) the art in question. (This does not exclude pleasure as one way of valuing art.) What is judged (dispassionately) here is the *value* (low or high) *as* artistry. Appreciation involves seeing what is bad about one artefact and relating that to what is good about another. It is possible, as Armstrong argues, to appreciate artistic failure (Armstrong, 1996, p. 21).

The question of who judges such matters is irrelevant. There is not one set of persons who can decide exclusively about such matters, it is the quality of the work that is to be judged, not the credentials of the person appreciating it that matter. What is important is the quality of the reasoning in the appreciation. This should be considered irrespective of matters of money, influence, advantage, or ideology. Equally, the *artistic* recognition of something is often quite separate from its *social* recognition. What gains popular (as opposed to professional) recognition depends on politics, propaganda and the power of the media. Appreciation, by contrast, is concerned with what is *there* to be recognized, whether or not it *is* so recognized (Armstrong, 1996, p. 24).

The appropriate reasons for valuing an object or process have to be related to what it is being valued as. (A pottery mug received as a present might be valued as a love token, an artefact or a drinking vessel.) Thus what the art is being valued as, is the crux of the matter of art appreciation. Pure art can, for example, be valued as an investment, or because of its provenance, or because of the prior fame of its creator, or *as a work of art.* Where it is valued *as art,* then we know more clearly what is relevant to valuing it in this way.

The 'best sort of criticism', as Armstrong points out, 'does not seek to set out *rules* for appreciation, or about what makes a painting artistically excellent; rather, it aims to bring to our attention what is fine about a particular work and to develop our capacity to appreciate: not judging for us, but enabling us to judge for ourselves' (Armstrong, 1996, p. 28). But such judgement, being an aspect of the discerning eye, needs to be carefully developed.

Thus, seeing – developing a discerning eye and an appreciative cast of mind – so as to receive and respond to the overall impact of professional artistry, is very complex. It would seem to involve:

- understanding the context (the history, traditions and physical context) within which the practice is carried out;
- discerning beneath professional practice the professional's aims, intentions and above all the professional's vision;
- being clear about the moral ends of the practice and the appropriateness of the means to these;
- being aware of the worth of the practice as professional practice;
- recognizing the professional's skills, capacities and abilities, theories, values, emotions, beliefs and personal qualities;

- seeing the artistic nature of the performance and perceiving what the professional has done to achieve artistry in respect of this;
- discerning in it the fusion (the balance and harmony, integration and unity) of the visible; together with the invisible (skills, thoughts, theories, values, abilities, emotions and personal qualities) and thus discerning the value of the practice *as a whole*;
- identifying the employment of imagination within the practice;
- distinguishing and distilling out from this picture the observer's own vision.

Armstrong says of visual art: 'At its greatest painting can condense a vision of the world and the loves of a lifetime into a perpetual object which communicates these to others' (Armstrong, 1996, p. 73). It might be said of professional artistry that at its very best it can imaginatively fuse a practitioner's vision, skills, capacities, abilities and personal qualities in such a way that they respond to the specific demands of a particular professional event, and create with originality *in* that event something of enduring meaning which can irrevocably shape for the better the life (and even the life chances) of the client (or pupils) involved. A key difference in all this, between pure art and professional artistry, is that the latter is far more ephemeral than a painting, being a process which happens at a specific time and within a specific time limit and which, once over, is as a process gone forever, but whose memory lingers and whose meaning ramifies. It is therefore, in this respect, more like an 'electrifying' performance in the theatre. But, like such a performance, it can be captured on film and/or recaptured (and then written about) on paper.

In the light of all this it is hardly surprising that the ability to appreciate practice in this way needs to be acquired. One means of beginning to acquire it is to set about witnessing and then considering the impact of a range of professional practice, and then to conduct a small investigation into one's own practice. An appropriate framework for such an exploration is case study, as is demonstrated below.

Case study research

Its appropriateness for investigating professional artistry

Golby, in a particularly useful text on the use of case study in research, argues that 'case study, properly conceived, is uniquely appropriate as a form of educational research for practitioners to conduct because it has potential to relate theory and practice' and can 'advance professional knowledge' by academically respectable means (Golby, 1993, p. 3). Indeed, he argues that it is 'synonymous with professional activity; it is what professionals do day by day' (Golby, 1993, p. 11). He also points out that 'the hall-mark of case study is not having a body of knowledge' about practice but knowing how to access the knowledge necessary to enlighten particular cases. But, he warns, 'case study is too often misconceived', and it is therefore important to understand the rationale for it (Golby, 1993, p. 3). Case study research is aimed at understanding practice in all its complexity and sees practice as part of the history and as shaped by the traditions of the practice of a profession. Case study research thus places emphasis upon reflection and deliberation, on context and meaning.

Other possible useful approaches are: illuminative enquiry, which focuses on the social world of practice, placing emphasis on data collection in community settings and being interested in illuminating these; and action research, which seeks from the outset to change practice and places emphasis on present data and theories of change, thus being more interested in a radical intervention than in understanding the present and its traditions and the potential for change from within. However, case study research is perhaps the most appropriate for appreciating practice. It should also be noted carefully that case study *research* is quite separate from and should not be confused with either 'clinical case study' (a study of a clinical case), or with taking or exploring a patient's case history (which is part of clinical practice).

Golby says the following of case study research.

- It advances professional knowledge by academic means.
- It offers the means of recording empirical investigations of contemporary real-life events.
- Case study is *not* the name of a method – there are many pos-

sible methods within case study research – but it is an overall approach to research within which specific methods may be selected on the basis of what the study of that particular case needs. Such methods will need to take account of the traditions from which they are drawn.

- Case study is appropriate where it is not yet clear what are the 'right' questions to ask.
- The case being studied must be a case of something seen in relation to wider ideas.
- You need to ask why you are studying it.
- It deals with *the particular* (not the unique). It is concerned with the particular seen as an example of the general.
- Premature closure is inimical to case study (see Golby, 1993).

Case study is also a particularly appropriate form for studying artistry in professional practice because, as MacDonald and Walker argue:

> case study is the way of the artist, who achieves greatness when, through the portrayal of a single instance locked in time and circumstances, he communicates enduring truths about the human condition. (MacDonald and Walker, 1977, p. 182)

This makes the point that though it is small scale, a case study, like a short poem, or a life-like portrait, can carry important truths.

Case study: a framework for the study of professional artistry

Case study involves a small scale enquiry by the enquirer into his or her own practice, and is useful at all stages of a professional's development. It takes as its focus a clearly bounded subject (person, institution, set of operations, professional problem) and catches its *particularity* and its *whole human complexity*. It is also possible to string several of these together to catch a set of complexities at another level. Case studies are 'strong in reality'; they are complex, messy, at times contradictory, yet these accounts can make telling connections within practitioners' experiences. It is, Golby argues, 'appropriate where it is not yet clear what are the right questions to ask', but where there is a sense of perplexity, problems to be addressed and a sense of a researcher's interest in those problems. A case, he suggests, 'must always be a case, or example, of something' seen in relation to a wider set of ideas. It starts from a provisional understanding and investigates it further (see Golby, 1993, pp. 5–6). It is not a study of uniqueness but of particularity.

A *framework for shaping a critical case study of professional artistry*

The following are the likely constituents of the process of producing a case study of professional artistry in which a portrait of practice and a critical commentary are key components. They are *not* entirely discrete processes. Chapter numbers in brackets indicate where further details are to be found.

The homing-in process (as found in this chapter)

- Explore a range of practice and of professional artistry, allowing it to make an impact upon you, and recording both the overall impression made and the reasons for the impact.
- Consider carefully what you are learning from these about both professional practice and artistry.
- Identify an issue or aspect of *personal* practice in which artistry seems to be evident and which would benefit from further scrutiny.
- Reflect on aspects and issues with a view to identifying *why and for whom* they are important.
- Consider and assemble the contextual information which will be necessary for understanding this practice.
- Deliberate about the issues raised when professional practice is appreciated in this way.

Produce draft portraits (see Chapter 9)

- Capture on paper – *briefly,* but as vividly as possible – a number of draft portraits of practice which are *illustrative of* professional artistry.
- Capture the contextual information which will be necessary for understanding this practice (produce a draft contextual analysis – clarify the context and consider critically both it *and the values implicit in the construction*).
- Consider and deal with explicitly in whatever way seems appropriate all those aspects of practice beneath its surface.

- Take account of own personal beliefs, values, perspectives as part of producing the portrait.
- Identify and deliberate about the *nature* of the professional artistry and what remains to be investigated.

Produce the final version of the portrait (see Chapter 10)

- Work to make this a holistic portrait.
- Work to utilize figurative language and artistic techniques and style in order to articulate those aspects of practice which are most difficult to explain.
- Highlight the details of the portrait by artistic means.

Investigate and produce a critical commentary on the portrait and the practice (see Chapter 11)

- Explore theoretical perspectives
  personal theory
  relevant formal theory
  overall parameters.
- Explore own on-going practice.
- Make meaning out of the problem, its context, the investigations and the values.
- Plan for the future.

9

Practitioner researcher as artist: working on draft presentations of professional artistry

Introduction

The intention of this chapter is to support colleagues as they attempt to produce draft portraits (narratives in words) of examples of professional artistry and seek to reflect upon those drafts and deliberate over the issues raised. By this means they will prepare for the production of the final version of a portrait of practice focusing on professional artistry or a specially chosen aspect of it (which will be discussed in Chapter 10). The drafts, and the reflections and deliberations which they provoke, might best be collected as the contents of a kind of artist's sketchbook or portfolio as described in Chapter 8.

It will quickly be evident that the processes here are creative ones and that the practitioner researcher has changed roles from artist practitioner to researcher as artist. By beginning this practical work the researcher begins fully to enter into the traditions of art which shape the thinking in this paradigm. This chapter is dedicated to supporting the adjustments that this requires of professionals for whom the science and the social science paradigms offer the more usual context for investigative work. (For example, we have already noted in Chapter 5 that research in the artistic paradigm cannot be designed and pre-planned in the same way as that in the other two paradigms. This means that practitioner researchers will need to adjust to working by 'feeling their way' towards broad goals and creating ways of operating in situ by responding to situations as they arise, as indeed they already do as art-ful practitioners.)

Entering into the traditions of the artistic paradigm does *not* mean however (as we shall see in detail below) that a researcher will need to be able to create 'real' art (quality fiction or quality paintings). What is necessary is having an interest in artistry, being willing to learn to *think like* – or more like – an artist, and being prepared to attempt various portrayals of practice (which themselves are artistic investigations). Since these portraits of practice will be *in words,* researchers will already be familiar with the medium (and indeed, were they researching in the interpretative paradigm, they would also be producing something which sought to capture practice – though perhaps normally with far less consciousness of the means available for in-depth, vivid presentation). The quality of the portrayals *as art* is not relevant here. The quality of the insights they offer and what such activities have enabled researchers to learn and to understand across a number of drafts are all that matter. The artist's workbook, sketchbook or portfolio used by the researcher to contain the basic evidence of such development, and the critical commentary on it, will provide the means of demonstrating this.

In order to support this work, this chapter falls into two main sections. The first is focused upon the new role of the practitioner researcher as artist, and the second section indicates and discusses the overall activities involved in the production of the drafts, and the concomitant reflection and deliberation on those drafts. It should be noted that the *production* of draft portraits – narratives – and the *processes of reflection on and deliberation about* them are in fact virtually inextricable, and will need to be captured as they occur (although they have here to be discussed separately for the sake of clarity). This is why the drafts and the thinking about them both need to be carefully preserved, and why an artist's portfolio or notebook/sketchbook is an appropriate means of collecting them. The chapter ends with a summary of the key practical processes which have been discussed.

Entering artistic traditions and taking up artistic processes

The two main sections of this chapter, then, offer ways of thinking about the artistry involved in the research process itself and particularly the procedures of producing artistic drafts. Such drafts attempt to capture various pieces of professional artistry so that their essence as well as their factual elements, the theories that underlie practice and the spirit of the practice, as well as the actions involved, are clearly articulated and presented. This will be a matter of making various sketches or attempts in words to capture and represent that professional practice which has made an impact on the researcher. The sketching process *itself* enables the researcher to discover why the subject has made its initial impact and to enable it to make further impact, as well as to refine (or to learn from) these attempts. And it should be remembered that a sketchbook often contains several attempts at sketching just one element of something, so that the painter can solve the problems inherent in depicting it, in order to be able to tackle a similar problem in a later painting. Key processes in that learning require a scrutiny of the drafts with a view to considering critically the artistry of professional practice, the artistry endemic in the research itself, and the evaluation of the potential of the paradigm.

This process might well uncover the need to acquire a little more knowledge and to develop further both understanding and technique before embarking on (or working one sketch into) the final portrayal. Practitioner researchers might need to go back again to the scene portrayed in order to learn more about the context, they might need to withdraw to think through some ideas, or to consult some relevant formal theory. The process will also reveal the impossibility of disentangling some elements of artistry, as well as some need to develop further representational techniques. However, it should be realized that rushing off to collect additional *data* because data is important to prove a point, is a notion endemic to empiricism (and implies a false relationship between 'researching' and writing it up). In fact (once the elements of the scene are identified and isolated), engaging in the *practice* of portrayal of what is seen and is being explored, is what matters. Uncovering new knowledge and developing new understandings and new techniques are, in the world of the Arts, *part* of the creative process, and will mostly occur not as a result of collecting yet more material, but *during* the production of both drafts and the final version. The portrayal of practice is not an exact factual matter, but rather is about catching the spirit. The artist is not a photographer, the novelist is not a scientist. Scientists and photographers deal with different *sorts* of truth from those that are revealed in painting or literature.

Thus, this work of producing draft portrayals of professional practice and of reflection on them and deliberating about the issues and truths they reveal (which, during the process of research in other paradigms, is of a kind often regarded as rough working to be scrapped once the work has been finalized) is an indispensable part of the creative process. Making drafts is what enables a writer to achieve the one that finally pleases best. And it should be noted that the draft chosen as the basis of the final portrait may not be the one produced last of all. Further, some elements from earlier drafts are often worth incorporating in the final portrait, and all drafts can provide important learning experiences. They will certainly provide (for discussion in the critical commentary) important evidence of the development of the discerning eye, the artistry of professional practice, and the artistry of the research.

The role of the artist researcher

Why is it even appropriate for a professional who wishes to investigate his or her practice to take on the role of artist researcher? The answer will need to refer to more than just the need to respond to artistry in the practice under scrutiny, since that might be achieved by a critic or connoisseur of professional practice. Surely (whatever kind of art is engaged in) the real reasons for trying to adopt an artist's viewpoint and activities is to grasp the distinctive character of the artist's job and of the particular cast of the artist's mind. It enables the researcher (like the artist) to be able to offer some vision of an aspect of the world which cannot be offered in any other way. That is, it is the opportunity to harness artistic perception, techniques and abilities and through them to depict the world in special ways, that the researcher gains from working within the artistic paradigm. And once the possibilities available to artists are understood, artist researchers will be able to adopt directly many of their techniques for use in capturing present professional practice. The success of such work *as art* is not of significance. It is its ability to help us see, share and consider practice in new ways that is so enriching. What then does an artist do? Wherein lie these special ways?

What is involved in working like an artist?

Artists are said to be able to 'open the eyes of others' to seeing aspects of the world anew, enabling them to recognize and search out details that they would otherwise miss (see, for example, Armstrong, 1996, p. 77). In literature such detail may be about manners and morals, character and motive as well as about the physical world itself. In much painting it is usually about a vision of the physical world (which often reveals, of course, something of its spirit and emotion and other – normally invisible – influences which have shaped it).

Artists, then, provide others with the means of seeing, by recognizing, isolating and capturing interesting scenes and accentuating the detail of these such that their underlying characteristics become clear. Such accentuation is achieved through all kinds of techniques which enable overlooked contrasts to leap out, the audience's perception of colours to be enhanced, relationships otherwise unnoticed to be indicated, matters normally invisible to be made plain. By these means – by this artifice – the picture presents elements of the original subject so as to emphasize them. In the words of Armstrong in relation to painting:

> In such ways the painter can draw our attention to features of the visible world which we in our haste and habit tend to miss; the painter does this not simply by noticing and recording, but by employing the resources of the art-form to make such visible phenomena more apparent than they would otherwise be. (Armstrong, 1996, pp. 77–78)

Thus, as we saw above on pages 41–44, artifice, used to reveal what otherwise would go un-noticed by the audience or reader, is not dishonest, but rather is a vital aspect of an artist's repertoire. Armstrong offers as an example of this the great play that the Impressionists made of the colours of shadows, saying: 'what happens is that the colour of shadows is made into a theme in the pictures, so that the eye is drawn to them more than it would be in reality' (Armstrong, 1996, p. 78).

Why does it take an artist (or someone who works like an artist) to do these things?

Of course is does *not* necessarily take an *artist* to notice such things or even to make them evident to others (it could be done by a scientist), but it takes an artist to make them 'tell artistically, to find in them material out of which a work of art could be made' (see Armstrong, 1996, p. 79) (my italics), and thus to be able to communicate some of the ineffable elements involved. Fortunately it is not necessary that such a person should be a great artist. As Armstrong points out, it is the achievement of the effect that matters not the ultimate value of the art. And this achievement involves not merely noticing details others might miss, but in uncovering the 'general quality of the scene, a general quality which does not fully reside in any particular detail' (Armstrong, 1996, p. 80).

As an example of this, readers are directed once more to the Bruegel painting. Here it is the overall impact of the painting which matters, and its distilling into that whole of a range of details (each one of which alone would not make anywhere near the same impression). The overall tone of the landscape, all the characters, and each little individual scene being enacted at different points on the canvas, all need to work together in order to make the entire picture. They create, of necessity *between them*, what the resources of the painter have been employed to show us. Armstrong offers the example of noticing that someone is a person who acts with tact, where it is the overall impression over a long period rather than a particular detail that has led to this judgement. Such observation is about noticing how, across time, they acted tactfully, and that the individual example of this only 'comes to be emotionally alive in the ensemble, precisely through its connection to other examples'. Many such 'diffuse qualities, which are not fully grasped in any particular detail' speak through a piece of art seen as a whole. (And it is for this reason that the paradigm proposed in Chapter 5 is referred to as the artistic/holistic paradigm.)

What artists offer their audience

Where scientific writing is to provide new knowledge for a specialist readership, by contrast, painters and literary writers present their work to stimulate the senses and the mind, and elicit the response to such stimulation of a wider group of people, who are usually thought of as an audience.

By enabling this audience *to see* and to sense the world more sharply and be aware of the gains involved, artists increase that audience's appetite for such sensory experiences, both in the world and through art, and they enable that audience to experience the fuller range of their own sensory powers. Thus, as Armstrong points out in relation to painting, the 'revelatory power' of art is not merely that it can show onlookers beauties, offer them some truths about beauty and lead them 'to a satisfaction where it would otherwise be unexpected', but that, at its best, art also reveals 'what perception can be'. The audience experiences this, as Armstrong argues, 'as a revelation', which 'does not so much reveal an empirical fact about the observable world: it yields a quality of experience' (Armstrong, 1996, p. 82). Such powers are available to practitioner researchers in helping themselves and others to become more aware of the impact of professional artistry.

Artists can open up such perception to an audience, and enable them to get closer to the ineffable and the mysterious, and allow them to come to grips with things of great importance to us all (like love, death and hope). Further, by means of encompassing the grandeur of 'great issues' in a single instance, artists can also utilize their techniques to enable an audience to see the subject of their work as a whole, including all the layers of meaning which lie under it. Art of all kinds thus provides a means of discerning – all at the same time – the many ideas, emotions, thoughts and values that run beneath any human action and activity. Again this is of considerable use to practitioner researchers in capturing and exploring the complexity of practice. It can also offer a means of capturing aspects of perceptual experience that are transient and normally elude our attention. Artists often achieve this (within the overall coherence of the work) by means of figurative language or expression which counterpoise contrasting elements such that they highlight the tension. For example, two opposites, or disparities (whether of image, idea, or character) can – in a painting or poem or novel – be held and caught in the amber of a vivid image as a still unity, when in the rush and tumble of life they are barely able to be articulated and are highly transient (see also Armstrong, 1996, p. 87).

But, of course, because they choose how they will depict a scene (and because such depiction can present things in ways that are not ever present in real life), artists can also control the way the audience sees. And the audience needs to be aware of this, and of artists' intentions, values, beliefs and attitudes towards their subject. These can be deduced from the treatment of the subject and the emotions which it evokes. It is important, therefore, to remember that art is not obliged to provide empirical 'truth', but can legitimately involve interpretation and exaggeration.

Working on these ideas: art does not yield to rules

It would be inimical to artistry (and more like painting by numbers) to attempt to indicate exactly how artist researchers might work on these ideas and how, in so doing, they might adopt the artistic techniques discussed at length in Part Two. But it is possible to indicate one framework of the kinds of overall processes that might be involved in operating in this way and which could be useful for exploring these ideas, and to offer some reminders of issues which will need attention within the drafts. The following sections, it is hoped, will both enable colleagues to experiment freely with and develop and consider critically these ideas, and to begin to home-in upon which elements of professional practice might best be worked upon further in order to be presented as a final portrait which will allow an aspect or aspects of professional artistry to be explored in detail.

Producing narratives of practice and reflecting and deliberating on them

Assuming that colleagues as practitioner researchers have already recognized an interesting subject (probably in their own practice), disentangled it from the generality of daily activity and isolated it in order to consider it further (as discussed in Chapter 6), this section considers four key processes. These are the representational task of depicting live practice; the processes involved in attending to the context of that practice in order to provide the necessary background for understanding it; the processes of seeing through the surface practice to what underlies it; and the activities of standing back and taking stock in order to reflect and deliberate on what has been achieved, what has been learnt and what more needs to be done. The following now looks at each of these in a little more detail.

Capturing live performance: impact and detail

Once a subject has been selected there is firstly the need to look carefully at the event to be depicted before finding ways of putting words on paper. (This is about re-viewing a live event, and may have to be done in your mind's eye if it has not been video-recorded. But even if it has been recorded it should be remembered that such a recording is itself an interpretation of, or one view of, what happened.) Look at this event in full and for some time. Only then is it important to make a start with words. When you do so, expect mistakes and the need to redraft or restructure, and treat these as learning points. Always remember that, like all professional practitioners, in entering your profession you have already proved your ability with words – both spoken and written. But also bear in mind that, as T. S. Eliot reminded us, 'words . . . slip, slide, perish, . . . will not stay in place, will not stay still' (Eliot, 1963, p. 194). This should mean that the task is approached with a useful mixture of self-confidence and humility!

The overall intention is likely to be of attempting to capture practice which is in some way illustrative of professional artistry, and of seeking, *as the words are put together*, to discover more about it and about artistry generally, and of offering this to an audience which has not witnessed it. The audience will need every help in seeing and sensing the multiple layers of events and in perceiving some truth about artistry as a result. In order to begin to achieve this, it will be important to experiment freely with a variety of kinds of drafts – even presenting the same piece in different ways, and getting some feedback from a critical friend.

The materials required to start this are no more than something to write with, some paper and some time with no other demands upon you, so that you can look back on a piece of practice in detail. What is *not* required is that you rush off first to collect lots of data! If time is short, then reduce the kind of sketch you can do accordingly, and keep it fairly simple. Start with something familiar and congenial and relatively small (like a critical incident of a piece of practice you believe was successful) and with a fairly simple intention of trying to re-capture the facts (about events but also about feelings), but at the same time try to present the general quality of the scene. Try to see it again. What impact did it make on you at the time and later? Why did it make this impact? What makes you want to present it on paper? Don't rush to write and to record what you see until you have thought about these matters.

Once you do put pen (or computer) to paper, be quick and bold to start with and seek to capture the spirit of the event – if necessary then fill in the details. Don't forget to date your work. What did you learn from this first attempt? Did you really look at your practice fully before you started to write or were you merely nursing an impression of what happened? (Looking properly, and perceiving fully is half the battle of most visual art. You may have to admit some failures here, but they are likely to encourage you to look more carefully in future.) Would it have been seen differently – recorded differently – by others involved? Is there a natural structure to what you have written? How does that compare with the structure of the original incident? Are there identifiable patterns in either, and if so what has caused them? If there are differences between the structure of the event and your presentation of it, why is this? (What is the difference between a record of an event and a presentation of an event?) Do you need to restructure the story so as to place the emphasis you want to convey more clearly? Could you tell this story from several differing points of view? Would it make different impacts as a result? Does the original impact bear up under closer scrutiny? Where are the essential elements of artistry in that practice? What characterizes them? What can be learnt about artistry here? Would all this be easier or harder to achieve if the practice described was not one's own?

Attending to the background: sketching the context

It will be important, as part of your sketch of a piece of practice, to paint the necessary background so that the subject (the particular piece of professional practice) can be properly understood in context. It is important here never to assume that your audience knows things which to you, the writer, are obvious. Ultimately, this will involve attending to three kinds of context (to look at the physical context, the historical one and to consider the traditions of practice which inform this particular piece). At this point in the proceedings the main need is to clarify the relevant physical context of the piece of practice (this may have been a natural part of the 'story' as you first told it, but even then you need to be sure that all the necessary contextual information has been provided, and if not, to provide more). How such information is obtained and then how it is infiltrated into the draft sketch will be a matter of professional judgement. It is likely to need to be incorporated at a redrafting stage, as is the following.

Seeing through to the theories: doing justice to the iceberg

It will be important to consider and deal explicitly with all those aspects that lie beneath the surface of the practice sketched. We referred to this in Fish and Coles as 'exposing and exploring that hidden realm of one's professional practice' (Fish and Coles, 1998, p. 305). There, we used the iceberg metaphor to encapsulate the idea that part of our practice (our professional 'doing' and 'saying') is above the surface and is visible (though we are often so busy about it that we do not stop to question it). But by comparison to the visible are the matters we described as 'below the water level' of the professional iceberg. These are 'our personal knowledge or "know-how" made up of personal theory, influenced of course by formal theory yet distinct from it too, our assumptions and expectations, our beliefs and values' (Fish and Coles, 1998, p. 305). Of these we noted that this aspect of our practice is hidden from view, hidden not just from others but from ourselves too. We added:

> the true expert, then, is someone who knows something of what lies beneath the surface of his or her practice, and spends time and effort not just understanding it but developing it further, and who can then talk about it more publicly too. (Fish and Coles, 1998, pp. 305–306)

These matters, then, need careful attention in any attempt to produce a vivid and insightful account of our practice. We particularly need to make reference to the personal theories that shape our work (theories-in-use) and those that we say shape our thinking (espoused theories) as well as that formal theory which we have internalized and utilized in practice, together with the assumptions, beliefs and values implicit in our actions. Again, how this is incorporated will be a matter of personal judgement in the light of what is seen as appropriate to the general quality of the scene as depicted.

Reflection and deliberation: standing back and taking stock

All artists stand back from their work from time to time during the process of creation. They do so in order to see what they have produced from another angle, and to reflect upon it and the processes involved in creating it. Similarly, it will be important to reflect upon the draft portrait and deliberate about the issues and truths it uncovers. During this process it will also be useful to take account of your own personal beliefs, values and perspectives as part of producing the portrait. Again, the help of a critical friend is worth enlisting. But don't fail to keep a record of this thinking, even where it involves talking aloud. The processes here are of two main kinds. That which is directed at refining the draft further (reflection on the success of the draft), and that which is concerned with the issues raised by it (reflection – and where possible deliberation – on the issues).

In terms of the first of these, the overall intention here is to identify the *nature* of the professional artistry depicted and what remains to be investigated. It will therefore be important to examine and appreciate in detail the nature of the practice and its artistry, as described in the draft. Does it, for example, do justice to the practice and your vision of that practice? Is it now possible to isolate the features which will need 'touching up' and highlighting in order to enable the audience to see what would otherwise go unnoticed? It is worth noting those aspects of practice which are particularly difficult to articulate, and considering how they might best be conveyed. Here is where further imagery or further detail might be necessary.

In terms of the issues raised by the draft, it will be important to consider the nature of the practice described and thus the kinds of questions it generates, to consider what other data will be needed before a final portrait can be drawn, to think critically about the practice, the context and your own interpretative role in producing the portrait, and to identify your own growth points in terms of understanding about artistry, professional practice and research.

Once these procedures have been completed, the artist researcher is ready to produce a final picture of practice or to work further upon one of the drafts already completed, as discussed in the following chapter.

A summary of the key processes discussed above

Working to produce draft portraits or narratives of practice

- Spend enough time looking at the practice to be sure that you have seen it properly.
- Capture on paper – *briefly,* but as vividly as possible – a number of draft portraits of practice which are *illustrative of* professional artistry.
- Capture the contextual information which will be necessary for understanding this practice (clarify the relevant physical context *and the values implicit in your construction of this context*).
- Consider and deal with explicitly, in whatever way seems appropriate all those aspects of practice beneath its surface.
- Take account of own personal beliefs, values, perspectives as part of producing the portrait.
- Identify the *nature* of the professional artistry and what remains to be investigated.

Reflecting upon the drafts and deliberating over the issues

Reflect upon the following, and where issues are debatable, deliberate over them, preferably with the help of a critical friend. Keep a record of this.

- Examine and appreciate in detail the nature of the practice and its artistry as described in the draft.
- Isolate the features which will need 'touching up' and highlighting.

- Note those aspects of practice which are particularly difficult to articulate, and consider how they might best be conveyed.
- Consider the nature of the practice described and thus the kinds of questions it generates.
- Consider what other data will be needed before a final portrait can be drawn.
- Think critically about the practice, the context and your own interpretative role in producing the portrait.
- Identify your own growth points in terms of understanding about artistry, professional practice and research.

10

Portrait of the professional as artist: finding a voice, developing a vision

Introduction

The intention of this chapter is to support the creation of a portrait of professional practice by an artist/writer, which will in some way have grown out of a desire to study professional artistry or some aspect of it (the artist/subject), and will have developed out of the practice of producing the kinds of drafts discussed in Chapter 8 (or will even have been selected from amongst such pieces for further development).

Such a portrait is likely to be a self-portrait (where the study will be autobiographical), although it may be a portrait of another professional and thus be biographical. For this reason, issues related to autobiography and biography as art are discussed below. But the main focus of this chapter is the production, by a professional, of a finalized picture of professional artistry at work. (This portrait will give expression to the performance of practice and to the invisible iceberg which underlies it.)

The intention, for the writer, behind the production of either self-portrait or portrait, is to provide a major means of developing and further exploring observation itself, depiction and appreciation. That is, the *process* of working on the portrait to finalize it, is itself a means of seeing that practice anew. This process involves seeing practice within the contexts which influence it, and discovering and making explicit the theorizing and the unrecognized beliefs and values which lie within the performance of practice or which are submerged elements within practice. It involves thinking critically about professional practice (and particularly its artistry) – at the level of both particular and individual example and general professional practice and principle. It is important to note that this is *not,* therefore, as is often implied in research in the interpretative paradigm, a matter of capturing what is an already preconceived and fully formed view of that practice.

As must by now be clear, for the purpose of investigation in the artistic/holistic paradigm (which is not about producing a major piece of art), the element of artistic *skills*, while it is of value, is of less significance than both the artist/writer's vision, and the techniques and resources which shape that vision and its presentation. Of these, it is *vision* – the artist/writer's ways of seeing – that is most important (see Langford, 1985, p. 9). Ways of seeing emerge – the final vision emerges – *only* during the final processes of production of the portrait. By contrast, obsession with technique is sterile and lacks vision (see Langford, 1985, p. 9). The critical commentary will be the place in which to discuss how well the vision has emerged and been conveyed through the skills available, to offer a further view of the vision, to relate it further to the wider professional context and literature and to consider what implications it has for the development of (personal) professional practice. These matters are dealt with in the following chapter.

Accordingly, this chapter concerns itself with how the portrait can be made to bring to light various aspects of the artist/subject's invisible iceberg of practice and how this can emerge during the process in which the artist/writer finds a voice through which to present the portrait.

For the purpose of this chapter, it is assumed that the final subject has already been selected for detailed presentation from amongst the drafts and has been reflected upon and deliberated about so that the iceberg and vision have already *begun* to emerge. It is also assumed that the key elements which need to be added to or refined within the picture of practice have been identified and that any final preparations for extending the content (involving the collection of further ideas and information) have been completed.

Working on the final draft will involve the artist/writer in seeking to find his or her own voice *during* the course of touching up the picture. It also involves ensuring that the final version offers an audience a clearer view of those new ways of seeing professional artistry which the artist/writer is discovering and seeking to convey. This will include pointing up themes, issues, queries, problems, and the theorizing of practice, and expressing a little more vividly those elements which, not being empirical, are unable to be described factually, as well as shaping and structuring the final work so that its written style carries the content in the most appropriate way and its overall composition underpins its unity.

This work also involves the exercise of discipline and control in respect of how much it is appropriate to alter the picture (in the light of the vision that the writer is seeking to present), and how far such alterations would achieve the improvement of that presentation (in artistic research and professional development terms). Knowing when to stop is important, as is keeping in mind the professional rather than the therapeutic nature of the investigation. Further, there is a need for the artist/writer to consider carefully his or her own changing relationship with the original subject (as a result of the finalizing process), his or her developing relationship with the audience, and the relationship of audience to portrait. It will be important to remember that in the end the audience will be in a position to validate (or otherwise) the artist/writer's work by whether or not they recognize it as a genuine picture of professional practice as they know it. Finally, to ensure the quality of the professional research and development, the rigour of the work is vital. This, in the artistic/holistic paradigm, depends upon the openness and honesty with which the nature and detail of practice 'comes off the page' and the integrity of the words used to convey it. (The rigour, as we discovered during the project reported in Fish and Coles, 1998, is *in* the writing.)

The following offers some comments on these matters in three main sections. The first section offers some comments on autobiography as seen in terms of art. The second is concerned with what is involved in the artist/writer finding a voice (establishing and stabilizing his or her own individual style and expression). This looks at some principles about: how and where to use accentuation in order to point up themes, ideas, images; ways of expressing the ineffable; and techniques for enabling structure to emerge from the writing in order to shape the whole into a unified composition. The third section looks at the relationships between subject, writer and audience.

The comments and suggestions in this chapter draw extensively on personal experience of attempting to portray practice – and practice settings – in various kinds of research (see, for example, the practice described in Fish, Twinn and Purr, 1990, and the vignettes in Fish and Purr, 1991). It also looks back on many years of work in supporting undergraduates and research students in education and health care as they sought to write about their own practice as part of various kinds of dissertations. But most particularly it is informed by the recent processes of supporting (and editing) the work of colleagues in education who wrote about their activities as tutors in initial teacher education (Fish, 1995b) and that of colleagues across a range of health fields as they refined their presentations of practice characterizable as artistry for Fish and Coles (1998). All this work has of course been conducted within the bounds of the interpretative paradigm, and mostly using case study, though as it has developed so the opportunities have increased for stretching the interpretative paradigm more in the direction of artistry. Indeed, cumulatively, it has produced overwhelming evidence for the necessity of an artistic paradigm.

Autobiography as art

Professionals are as they are and work as they do because of their personalities and previous histories. This is why autobiography makes an important contribution to professional development. As noted in Fish and Coles (1998, p. 214), much has already been written of the contribution of autobiography to reflective research and its uses in humanistic enquiry (for example: by Abbs; Boud, Keogh and Walker; Grumet; Pinar and Woods). But in professional literature it is less often remembered that both biography and autobiography were first of all art forms in themselves, whose roots may be traced back to the seventeenth century (see Fish and Coles, 1998, pp. 214–218, for details).

What then is involved in the artistic creation or enhancement of portraits of professional practice? How does vision emerge as the writer finds his or her voice? Firstly, it involves recognizing that autobiography is a proper form for this work and that the use of the personal pronoun being a sign of this, it should neither be expunged from the portraits nor replaced by more formal and impersonal modes of expression. Further, the writing should not be sanitized of its inevitable subjectivities and informalities. This work is in the artistic/holistic paradigm, and such matters are a central part of this location. Indeed, the need for the artist/writer to find his or her individual voice in order to enable the full significance of the portrait to be presented, is itself a signal that these matters need to be accentuated rather than obliterated.

The importance of voice

The formal voice of writing

In most research, and even much writing which is focused upon professional issues, the voice used is an adopted one of formal, professional and scholarly neutrality. It is intended to convey the idea that this work is objective, unbiased, cool, deliberative – and thus reliable. Most professional journals still require it, irrespective of the intention, focus and subject of an article. And writers expect to provide it. As a result of this they often spend much time creating what can only be described as a highly artificial voice. They seek to 'improve' (sanitize) their original draft by expunging its individual character. They replace the words that give away attitudes and emotions with tempered phrases, they exchange emotive language for measured tones. They also substitute the impersonal third person for the first person wherever it has crept in by mistake, or rewrite to insert longer sentences which allow them to avoid referring to any person at all. They reduce what could be the beginnings of a rich description to what they (misguidedly) think of as 'pure' fact. They embark on complex clauses and lengthy sub-clauses to ensure the greatest possible accuracy of expression (and sometimes trip themselves up as a result). They strive to present abstract arguments full of self-conscious logic but empty of human life. And even when it is clear that doing all this distorts the content and intention of their writing, they rarely rebel (but instead withdraw the article and accept the implied failure). Indeed, the power of publishers and of editors both as censors of, and shapers of, critical discourse today is frightening! This is, too, striking evidence of the grip in which positivism holds us all. It is the result of being brought up to believe that all publishable writing about serious matters in professions requires a standard scientific approach. It reveals just how unaware we are of the enslavement we are in. And at base, it shows a total ignorance of the importance, in all writing, of voice.

Voice in literature

By reference to a wide range of literature, culminating in a reference to the apocalyptic voices of The Book of Revelation at the end of the Bible (where the voice is described as being like music, a lion and thunder, and is presented in terms of many voices, including that of prophecy), Bennett and Royle claim that:

> literature, in fact, might be defined as being the space in which, more than anywhere else, the power, beauty and strangeness of the voice is both evoked or bodied forth *and* described, talked about, analysed. In this respect, reading literary texts involves hearing extraordinary voices. (Bennett and Royle, 1995, p. 59)

Successful writing depends greatly on creating a voice which is appropriate to the writer, the subject and the intentions of the work. Voice is the means of carrying content. Writers need to enable their audience to place the voice of their writing, and readers need to be able to recognize, through hearing the voice, the writer's emotions about and attitude to self, subject and audience. It is tone of voice which tells an audience how to interpret what is being conveyed – whether it is intended to be comic, satiric, sad, thoughtful – and which thus gives an audience a starting point from which to respond. Voice is created through vocabulary, subject reference points, use of tense and person of verb, repetition, use of figurative language, tone, emphasis, transcribed pronunciation. It conveys much about the writer beyond what the writer is saying – or, put another way, it offers a further context in which to place and through which to understand what is conveyed in words. It can convey highly significant matters like age, gender, experience of life and topic.

Writers have the opportunity to create a voice which is different from their own (in Bennett and Royle's terms : 'to make an implicit distinction between narrator and author'). This even enables a writer to handle individual and particular events and activities (in one voice) against a background commentary of general issues to which it is in special ways related (in another voice). Indeed, where a portrait of practice is integrated with a critical commentary upon it (as happens even in interpretative paradigm research), this is the technique actually being used. (But *there* it is mostly being used without the consciousness which would allow its use to be improved.) From this we can begin to see that 'a question of voice is never simple, even (or perhaps especially) when it appears to be' (Bennett and Royle, 1995, p. 63). It is worth noting that texts can also say things directly about voice and how the reader should hear it, and that there is almost always more than one voice in a literary text ('even if it is just talking or responding to itself') (Bennett and Royle, 1995, p. 63). Indeed, it is possible that there is no such thing as a single (simple) voice, but that there is multiplicity within every voice.

What is called 'voice' in literature is referred to as style and expression in painting. In both, it is possible to talk about the voice or style (even tradition) of a period or a genre. At the level of an individual who embarks on a piece of writing, however, a writer stamps personality on events and creates a voice for himself or herself (but only insofar as current traditions allow, because – except for great innovators – his or her way of seeing the world is shaped by those traditions). Voice then is a major means of conveying vision. When we speak of a novelist or poet being distinguished by his or her own voice, we are referring to that which reflects (within the resources generally available at the time of writing) his or her particular mode of sensibility, attitudes towards characters, events, moral complexities and reader. And such a voice will be characterized by preferred figurative language, sentence structure and cadence, as well as his or her particular solution to the problem of controlling a body of imaginative material 'which must emerge with the imprint of a unified view of life' – like the overall shape of paragraphs and sections and the ultimate composition (see Ginger, 1970, p. 105).

In relation to an individual painter, style refers to the techniques and practices which govern all aspects of how his or her painting looks. A set of practices and devices which are experienced as having a high degree of consistency, govern *how* the picture is made (see Armstrong, 1996, p. 98). He says:

> when a particular painter in his own work gradually pieces together a complete and coherent set of techniques and guides which suit his own aesthetic purposes, then we say that he has developed a personal style. Others who are influenced by his work can take up this

set of techniques. In so doing, they are adopting a general style: something they did not discover for themselves and which others too may adopt. (Armstrong, 1996, p. 98)

Armstrong also makes the point that (in both painting and literature) personal style can be a vehicle for expressing personality more than anything else (Armstrong, 1996, p. 99).

It is, of course, possible in art of all kinds to adopt someone else's voice, to take over wholesale and/or mimic the style and expression of another writer as well as to 'become another character'. And indeed, some people advocate imitating other writers as a kind of apprenticeship to writing (with the intention of gradually shedding this in favour of a style that is individual). This is one means of starting to be creative within a sheltered structure. On the other hand, it is not conducive to the emergence and ownership of the vision enshrined in the writing.

Finding a voice, developing a vision

In seeking to discover congenial ways of solving the problems of how to accentuate a particular effect, idea, or issue, then (as well as how best to express the ineffable, how to pull the writing together into a unity which works at all levels, and yet operate in a controlled and disciplined way), artist/writers will be seeking the *emergence* of their own natural style – their own guidelines, techniques and practices. These, of course, cannot be rule-governed. All that can be offered in support of this is some principles which might provide guidance.

Accentuating themes

Whether the artist/writer is attempting to produce a visually vivid scene, to diffuse the entire occasion with a particular emotion and tone, or to highlight or simply exaggerate or suppress one small vivid detail, the principles are the same. Artifice is what is involved – yet it is artifice employed with a view to producing, revealing or discovering a deeper truth about the subject. And this is where the artist/writers become researchers who seek artistic truth – truth which, for all its subjectivities, is concerned with issues which lie at the heart of the human condition (where scientific truth, with its concern for objectivity, is concerned more with the visible surface of our lives). The artist/writer's task here is not merely about expressing an individual and highly personal vision, though the temperament and personality of the artist will govern selection and preference. Rather it is about the results of:

> a way of seeing [which] makes it possible not only to see things as they are but also to construct a vision of how they might be, a vision which in turn is changed into reality by the painter's [writer's] activity. (Langford, 1985, p. 18)

The task of the writer, then, is to develop a vision of the subject by reviewing a piece of writing and seeking in it the underlying ideas, emotions, significance, as a first step in attempting to highlight its underlying character. This is likely to involve the use of greater emphasis, or simplification, or selection and suppression, or exaggeration, in order to make the vision in the writing clearer and thus more available to readers. Eisner, following Ryle, called this 'thick description' (Eisner, 1979, p. 195). The artist/writer, like the painter described by Armstrong, needs to seek to provide a compelling visual image in which writer and audience can see or sense a key idea which is not usually visibly present to them. This can also involve simplifying the sentence structure in order to allow the contrast to stand out.

Highlighting gets rid of stock description and stock response. It is about accentuating contrasts, either by adding more of the medium used, or removing some. For example, the painter of life studies is well aware of and often reveals to the audience, the skeletal structure beneath the flesh he or she is depicting. By adding a shadow here and by lifting paint off there, that skeleton beneath the flesh is made clearer to us even though no naked bone has been painted. Making one thing stand out is itself a means of reducing the significance of another. And in the written word there are many devices for this. They do not have to be sophisticated devices in order to be highly successful. For example, the sudden vivid image, the switch to a more direct and personal address to the reader, the use of headings and subheadings, and the careful placing within a paragraph of important matters all conduce to this end. And much of the hidden iceberg of professional practice can be pointed up and examined by these means. Indeed, the usefulness of this metaphor is itself a further indication of the power of images.

It is sometimes instructive to look through a piece of writing and discover how many such devices one has already used subconsciously. Some of these might then benefit from being given greater emphasis, perhaps to make them more available for the reader. But it should, of course, be remembered that if contrast is to achieve its potential there needs to be a slight element of surprise with it, and this is not obtained, and certainly does not allow a vision and understanding of practice to emerge, if it is *imposed* on a piece of writing at regular and predictable intervals rather than emerging from and underpinning the ideas presented in the portrait.

One key means of accentuation, which is also invaluable in conveying the ineffable in practice, is figurative language.

Expressing the ineffable

The ineffable and mysterious elements in professional practice are best identified as well as best expressed through figurative language. (This term is used to cover everything from metaphor, metonymy and simile to personification, hyperbole and anthropomorphism, as well as symbolism and allegory.) In fact all our written and spoken language is figurative, but we have become so accustomed to some of the more common usages that we no longer notice them. A writer's job is to keep the language fresh so that it opens readers' eyes to the text. It is vital to avoid tired ways of saying things. The manipulation of figurative language has fundamental implications for the way we understand the world (as we see daily in the news media). As Bennett and Royle point out, 'the meaning of a text cannot be separated from its expression, its figures' (Bennett and Royle, 1995, p. 67).

In the context of producing a portrait of practice, figurative language is not about providing added-on ornament, but is useful for communicating or stimulating insight. It is less about prettifying visible matters already conveyed, than about expressing the ineffable which has not yet been captured. In all cases, it will only be successful if it emerges from the content rather than being imposed upon it. The term 'ineffable' here is not meant to refer to those matters encapsulated in the metaphor 'hidden iceberg of practice', because many of these are merely subconscious matters which once brought to the surface can be discussed in fairly literal and concrete terms, and which can be accentuated as indicated above. Rather it is used here to describe those elements of practice which are hard to sense, are hard to capture in any simple concrete description. This might be because they are nuances or fleeting thoughts and feelings, mere tinges on solider colours, or because so many things are happening at once during a particular incident (or because ideas are needing to be held together in an overall unity) that there are matters which cannot be grasped and conveyed by simple, chronological description. As poets have always known, an image, by contrast to more pedestrian description can convey a complicated mixture of vision, emotion and idea *in one instant*.

Aristotle talked of metaphor as a process rather than a commodity, as a mode of perception rather than an object (see Ruthven, 1969, p. 5). Metaphor and simile, particularly, are about perceiving and pointing up a similarity of ideas, by first recognizing an association between apparently unlike images and then yoking them together in a vivid phrase which startles the reader into reconsidering their relationship. (Examples of this are quoted in abundance in Chapter 3, where we see writers likening professional practice to elements of the arts, and also in Chinn and Watson, 1994, and in *Educational Theory,* volume 45, number 1.) Equally, in the hands of poets, such figures of speech can make the apparently concrete *less* visible or imaginable, can disturb our normal understandings, can merge the figurative and the literal, and can turn ideas reflexively back on themselves.

At its best, the careful use of figurative language by the artist/writer can enable several ideas to be entertained together by the reader in the same moment. Indeed, the hidden iceberg of practice is a good example and enables readers to see and to think anew. Figurative language is uniquely able to help us grasp in a single instance some of the more difficult ideas, emotions, moral complexities endemic to professional practice, and to see as a whole a number of layers of meaning. It can also offer a means of capturing aspects of perceptual experience that are normally transient, or elude our attention and are barely able to be articulated. Writers often achieve these things by means of counterpoising, contrasting and using striking visual imagery such that they highlight the tension between similarity and dissimilarity. Such a counterpoising will ensure that the two opposites (whether of image, idea or character) are held together, unified in a vivid moment of stillness.

And sometimes writers, finding their images apt in expressing an idea, discover that the figure can be extended, though it is unwise to stretch any figure of speech beyond its ability to enable readers to gain fresh perceptions and insights from it.

At moments of dramatic or emotional intensity, figurative language tends to come to mind more frequently (or perhaps it is that life mimics literature here, for certainly in literature, figurative language seems to flow at such points). But, again, such figurative language is not added decoration, but is endemic to thinking and feeling. This is neatly caught in Bennett and Royle's comment that: 'an alteration in the way we figure the world also involves an alteration in the way that the world works' (Bennett and Royle, 1995, p. 67). They add, significantly for writers of professional portraits: 'Figurative language can make us see what is otherwise invisible' (see Bennett and Royle, 1995, p. 68). And an audience or reader can learn about a whole text by focusing on its figurative language. In this sense of course, figurative language which acts as a theme throughout a piece of writing can be one means of establishing its overall unity.

Enabling structure to emerge and working towards unity of composition

Just as during writing a voice needs to be found to convey the portrait, and the vision carried within the portrait has to emerge during its production, so its structure is also best discovered *during* the final writing, rather than being imposed upon it. But this is not the same as suggesting that the artist/writer should set out with no sense of structure. A literary text begins long before the words of the first paragraph of the final draft are written. In the case of the portrait, ideas which emerged during the practice itself and the early drafts will have shaped the overall structure on which the writer then embarks. But this may well change as the writing proceeds. And with the ability of the computer to move text around, there is every reason to continue to question the order and organization of a text right up until it has been printed in its final form.

In considering structure it is important to remember that the individual sentence is a key unit in writing of this kind, and that the structure of sentences carries tone, creates music and fits (or ill-suits) the content being conveyed. For this reason sentence structure is worth working on. Indeed, if it is long, it is often worth reducing in length and turning into two sentences. The principles here are about clarity of communication and about appropriateness of structure and form to content. Thus the same principles can be applied to paragraphs and sections. A careful system of headings and sub-headings can be useful for reader as well as writer. And it will be necessary to attend too to the overall sense of unity of the piece, again using the same principles as a basis. Here, it is important not to be tempted to impose a false unity on the portrait (for example by planting a number of images and themes which are drawn together at the end), but to work over the piece until its inherent unity emerges.

Writer, subject and audience

We noted in Fish and Coles (1998, pp. 215–216), that when we read autobiography we are juggling with several perspectives at once:

> the writer's original and immediate view of events, thoughts and feelings (including sometimes that writer's sense of how posterity might judge him or her), the reader's modern response to all this and, mixed up with it, the view the modern reader gains through the advantage of hindsight which by definition was not available to the writer.

This serves to alert us to the complexity of relationships between writer, subject and audience, which complexity the artist/writer needs to be aware of and to take account of while refining the portrait of practice.

Portrait and writer

At the point of finalizing the portrait (having made a decision that the work is complete) the artist/writer will have produced an end result which has been shaped by intention and which has emerged as a result of discovery. At this point it will become a public portrait, and will become the property of an audience. And it is possible for the audience to value a work of art quite differently from, and in ways that go beyond, the artist's original vision. A work of art has a multi-dimensional character and there is no one right way of deciphering it, although (despite modern fashion) the author will always be seen as some sort of authority about what he or she has created. And, of course, this will particularly be so in autobiographical work, where writer and subject are in a special relationship. Nevertheless, once the portrait is public property its significance will change for the artist/writer, and those matters that were private will be open to critical scrutiny.

In this case, it will be important to have heeded the warnings of Daedalus in Joyce's *Portrait of the Artist as a Young Man* (Joyce, 1967). In writing about self, where both emotional reactions to events and emotional involvement with subject threaten to be just a whisker away, the artist/writer needs to keep some emotional distance from subject, and to control the writing so that the audience too is allowed to remain equidistant emotionally. Otherwise, ironically, what will be unbearably significant and significantly unbearable for writer will be plainly unacceptable to audience. The process of progressive focusing involved in working through several drafts of the portrait crucially enables this to happen. In Fish and Coles (1998) we pointed out, in reference to the autobiographical work of our contributors, that what Joyce's hero says is highly relevant here. We summarized this as:

> the centre of emotional gravity needs to be equidistant from the artist and the audience. The narrative is no longer purely personal. The personality of the artist passes into it but becomes refined and impersonalized through subsequent drafts until the writing becomes transformed into a public work. (Fish and Coles, 1998, p. 247)

Art and the audience

What relationship, then, should an artist have with his or her audience? And what relationship should the audience have with the work of art itself? How should an audience respond to works of art? Perhaps the role of critical audience is both to seek to give a faithful response to the artist's vision and to take that vision and turn it into something new in their own professional lives by recognizing the work as part of a tradition, their response as part of the response of a critical community, and by creating a new vision out of it.

But, in the case of the work of the artist/writer working in a professional research and development context, there is the opportunity to shape this response by offering a critical commentary. And this, as we shall see in the following chapter, is where the professional practitioner using ideas from the Arts and appreciation of the Arts to enlighten practice, *unlike the artist,* can be a connoisseur and critic as well as a creator.

11

Deepening our appreciation of the artistry of practice: creating a critical commentary

Introduction: going deeper

In the earlier chapters of this part of the book we have recognized that appreciation is about cultivating a discerning eye and developing a particular cast of mind, and involves valuing artistry for appropriate reasons. We have seen that producing early drafts can provide opportunities to experiment in perceiving and describing practice and its artistry within an artistic/holistic paradigm – opportunities to enter more fully into artistic traditions and to take up artistic processes. And we have explored how finding a voice enables us to shape and finalize or crystallize and thus preserve a vivid portrait of practice. It now remains to add to what has already been accomplished by seeking to deepen the appreciation of that portrait and the practice which it presents, through the creation of a critical commentary which is attentive to the voice of the writer/artist, alert to the nature of professional practice and which is also concerned with the development of taste.

A critical commentary in the Arts is the means of thinking about a particular piece of art *as a whole* by responding to it holistically, and by seeing it in a broader context. The same process applies to appreciating professional practice and its artistry. Here consideration of the broader context enables us to relate the portrait and its subject to the traditions of practice of that profession, to the life of the professional, and to a range of professional considerations and their associated literature. Here, analysis, interpretation and evaluative judgement all have their part to play in considering the significance of the portrait and its subject, *as practice*, and in terms of professional artistry, and through this, in providing a vision for the future. It should be remembered too that the critic comes to this with his or her own vision and values, which also must be declared if the work is to be open to judgement by the audience.

In creating such a commentary, it should be remembered that it is entirely possible to gain much understanding about professional practice from a portrait of considerably less than high quality art which in turn captures relatively ordinary (though not trivial) practice. This is also true in painting. As Armstrong points out, 'some pictures do offer us finer and more profound things to appreciate than others'. He notes that:

> there must be as there are in all things which involve skill, a place for the recognition of acquired professional competence, which, while perhaps not achieving the heights, is far above the work of the amateur. This includes the sort of finesse which comes with experience. Such work offers a good deal to the appreciative eye: while not of the first rank it may still offer aesthetic satisfaction. (Armstrong, 1996, p. 142)

It is also important to note that taste, and the ability as well as the capacity to appreciate, need themselves to be developed (through practice in writing good critical commentaries). Armstrong points out that: 'as taste develops there is a tendency to home in on the greater things', but that the art critic's personal history of the development of appreciation will inevitably 'be made up of wide circuitous wanderings, false starts, backtracking and returns' (Armstrong, 1996, p. 127). Every attempt at producing such a commentary is itself a learning process, and as such needs to be shared with others – both critical friends and the wider audience of professional colleagues and public.

To the end of supporting colleagues who are attempting to create a critical commentary, this chapter is offered in two main sections. The first looks at issues related to the intentions of such commentaries. The second section looks at the starting points and main processes involved in creating such a critique. The conclusion then looks forward rather than back.

Responding to the whole picture: the nature of the critical commentary

The critical commentary here discussed is a full appreciation of the overall portrait of professional practice. Whether the portrait is autobiographical or biographical, the same principles and processes are relevant. In such a commentary a critic with an educated eye and an insider's knowledge of the subject matter and of the processes of creating such a portrait, stands back from what has been presented in order to look at it as a whole, and through it to consider critically and to learn about *professional practice and its artistry*. It should be remembered that the task of appreciation is an open-ended one. In order to elucidate the nature of such a piece of writing we shall consider its main intentions, we shall look at the role of the critic, and at what is involved in the capacity to appreciate.

The main intentions

A critical commentary seeks to focus on, and consider critically, significant elements of the painting or writing in question and to heighten and expand the audience's awareness of them. And in this it is inevitably subjective and evaluative and must be acknowledged as such. It is, as we noted above, the place in which to discuss how well the vision has emerged from the portrait and how well it has been conveyed through the skills available (and, if necessary, to offer a further view of the vision), to relate it further to the wider professional context and literature and to consider what implications it has for the development of (personal) professional practice. And, of course, the qualities described must be able to be located in the portrait itself (see Eisner, 1979, p. 191; also Armstrong, 1996, p. 20).

A critical commentary can both open up an exploration of more detail in the portrait and its subject (reflect more deeply), or, equally, move away from the text and deliberate upon the issues it raises. Clearly, good critical commentaries do both. And in both cases the starting point involves critical concepts being brought to bear upon the portrait itself. There can also be, of course, some unintended outcomes of a critical commentary, and some disappointments. It can, for example, if handled badly, say more about the commentator than the object of the commentary. Further, a work may be highly imaginative, and yet the critic may discover by attending to it that the experience which we are invited to have by the work is not one which we can regard as being of high artistic value (see Armstrong, 1996, p. 122).

The work of a critic in this respect is not easy. The portraitist has rendered the ineffable qualities of professional practice palpable through the use of figurative language. The critic must now render the same qualities 'into a language that will help others perceive the work and the practice more deeply'. Again, it is interesting how the texture of the very language used here to highlight this point becomes highly figurative in character in the attempt to express more difficult ideas. For example, Eisner points out that: 'In this sense the critic's task is to function as midwife to perception, to so talk about the qualities constituting the work of art that others, lacking the critic's connoisseurship, will be able to perceive that work more comprehensively' (Eisner, 1979, p. 191). On the other hand, for Dewey (as Eisner also points out) 'the end of criticism is the re-education of the perception of the work of art' and is about 'lifting the veils that keep the eyes from seeing' (see Eisner, 1979, p. 191). By contrast, in Fish and Coles (1998, p. 224) we said:

> we shall now attempt to open up the writing before you . . . and enable you to see . . . the significance below the surface and to discern the whispers of what lies just beyond its voiced details . . . . And in so doing we recognize and acknowledge our own subjectivities, values, assumptions, beliefs, interests.

Indeed, Chapters 12 and 13 of Fish and Coles (1998), which contain several perspectives on critical commentary, offer useful examples here. There, we ourselves produced the commentary on the portraits of practice offered by our contributors. We saw each portrait as a journey in the development of 'one practitioner's understanding of individual practice viewed from within the wider context of professional artistry and understood in terms of the wider traditions of health care and a particular health care profession' (Fish and Coles, 1998, p. 222). We recognized that we had been made privy to individual insights, and we made the point that by attending to their voices we were able to appreciate more fully what is being said and thus offer a critique of it.

In respect of producing a critical commentary on (a thoughtful and critical review of) the work of our six contributors, we said that our intentions were:

1   To respond – as active and discerning readers who are also reflective practitioners – to the printed word and through that to the ideas it enshrines about professional practice, to the wholeness of the individual chapters and the unity that they constitute (the integrity, harmony, balance, proportion and symmetry).
2   Whilst so doing, to give evidence of our reliability as honest and diligent critics, to treat the writers and their work with a proper respect and attend to the relationship which we develop with our (and their) readers.
3   To point to and thus to point out (indicate) the qualities of the writing, to nudge the reader to see links and patterns, and locate, recognize and probe the insights. (See Fish and Coles, 1998, pp. 209–210.)

We also argued that we sought not to offer our interpretation ('by imposing our admittedly subjective meanings on it in order to explain it') but instead to present what we believed was a thoughtful critical *response* which we produced by any and as many means as possible. We also accepted that 'there may always be more means to understanding it than have been operated and as many ways to appreciate it as there are human beings to do the appreciating'. And we claimed that so far as our inevitably subjective reading allowed, we tried 'to let its content and artistry speak for itself' (Fish and Coles, 1998, p. 223).

In much of the above it is impossible to distinguish totally between critical commentary and critic, and so the following takes up these ideas by looking at them from the critic's perspective.

Critics and their role

Eisner provides some perspectives on the role of the critic when he says: 'Criticism is the art of disclosing the qualities of events or objects that connoisseurship perceives'. Critics, he says, 'do not aspire toward a translation of an event . . . for it cannot be made', rather they give 'an account of an experience which is never a substitute for experience'. Perhaps with the subconscious image of the art critic standing in the art gallery in mind, Eisner says, of critics, 'they create a rendering of a situation or event or object that will provide pointers to those aspects of it that are in some way significant'. He makes the point, of course, that what counts as significant will depend upon theories, models, values and the purposes of the critic (see Eisner, 1979, p. 197).

The role of the critic then is crucial in enabling access to the work by a wider audience. Eisner argues, that the critic needs 'a lot of experience of [professional] practice to be able to distinguish what is significant about one set of practices or another' (Eisner, 1979, p. 211). Armstrong, talking of painting, argues that the finest critics:

> induce us into a mood of receptiveness, they foster in us the attitudes or excitements which are important if we are to see the point of certain work, if we are to have feeling for it. They encourage, as it may be, a love of stone and of the working of stone; they bring us as it were into the community in which we get the joke, or see the point. (Armstrong, 1996, pp. 134–135)

He adds a little later, 'they direct our eyes and attention in a situation which is unfamiliar' (Armstrong, 1996, p. 135). There is however, as he points out, an important distinction to be made between the quality of the picture and the quality of the enthusiast's relation to the picture (Armstrong, 1996, p. 128). But also, a good critic (like a good consultant) should work to become redundant. As Armstrong says (associating himself with the audience), in the end 'the features of a picture, like its gracefulness, delicacy, bold design, balance, are things which we want to see for ourselves' (Armstrong, 1996, p. 135).

As in all matters, the quality of the critic will determine the quality of the commentary, or as Eisner puts it: 'criticism can only be as rich as the critic's perceptions' (Eisner, 1979, p. 211). Thus, an ill-disciplined critic, for example, can read into a picture all manner of things which cannot be found anywhere at all in the original. And even where they can be found, he or she can ascribe to them meanings that are entirely personal. This should be avoided by recourse to the usual scholarly strategies in such matters, as discussed below. These matters of course also relate to the critic's – and the audience's – capacity to appreciate.

The capacity to appreciate

The capacities involved in appreciation are essentially open-ended, and are abilities that can be refined and developed over time. They cannot, like skills, be trained, or even taught. Rather, they are acquired (though a teacher – or in this case a critic – may act in a corrective role in relation to this). It is one thing to have capacities and another to be willing to exercise them (see Passmore, 1980, p. 38). For Eisner, the vital capacity for the critic is the ability 'to perceive what is subtle, complex and important'. For him, 'to be a connoisseur is to know how to look, to see and to appreciate . . . and, significantly, to recognize the way particulars form a whole structure, to be able to conceptualize the underlying structure and see it as an overall activity, to see it as a whole' (see Eisner, 1979, p. 191). He also notes that such recognition leads to classification, but that – in the end – *seeing* is the achievement. The development of the perception of subtleties comes with exploration driven by a desire to improve (see Eisner, 1979, p. 194).

Armstrong argues that we need imagination, sensuality and spirituality to look at paintings. In a memorable and significant sentence he says: 'Divested of imagination, practical good sense degenerates into routine and philistinism; separated from sensuality, intelligence grows cold; spirituality, cut off from understanding, is in danger of falling into eccentricity'. He argues that we should aim at a response to art which reintegrates these capacities which are so diverse in human nature, and that at best some paintings themselves have been able to achieve this (Armstrong, 1996, pp. 140–141).

Taste is a major capacity which the processes of appreciation seek to develop. In relation to tracing the process of how taste in painting develops, Armstrong offers ideas equally appropriate to the appreciation of artistry in professional practice. He notes that people come to have a more appreciative relation to the pictures they like by working to perceive them more fully both in terms of detail and as holistic entities. He argues that three capacities contribute to this: imaginative yearning ('our effort of re-creation, of imaginative exercise, of trying to make use of the impression and the feeling it arouses'); the role of others in leading the eyes, in cultivating the sense of what to look at and how to look; the grasp that a great work transcends private associations. In the absence of these capacities, he says, engagement with a painting is liable to be sterile (Armstrong, 1996, p. 132). He also notes that 'the growth in our capacity to appreciate is accompanied by a change in the object of interest' (Armstrong, 1996, p. 127). (As we become more discriminating we seek more sophisticated examples of good art or good practice.)

Given these intentions, and this kind of critic, who will be developing in himself or herself as well as in his or her audience the kinds of capacities here described, what are the main processes involved in creating a critical commentary?

Discerning the whispers beyond the voice: creating a critical commentary

This section looks at some starting points, and at the activities that are central to the production of a critical commentary, and also considers ways of ensuring reliability and validity, and justifying judgements.

Starting points

The beginning of a critical commentary must be with the object or objects of that commentary or with matters directly connected to these. (This means the portrait of practice and its original subject.) Here it is important to remember the advice also given about preparing to produce a portrait of practice. It is vital to let the subject (in this case the portrait and the practice it presents) make an impact, to give it time to work upon us. Appreciation comes by degrees. It is rather like looking at photographic paper in a developing tray and seeing the picture – or in this case the portrait, the practice and their full significance – emerge. And this applies whether or not the portrait is an autobiography, because once finalized it takes on a life of its own which needs to be recognized even by its original creator. As Armstrong points out in relation to paintings, 'In the first few minutes what an observer takes in depends largely on his or her perceptual history' (Armstrong, 1996, p. 115). He also points out that 'there are relations between the parts of the picture which have to be digested slowly' and that it takes time to grasp what a picture really looks like (Armstrong, 1996, p. 115). He says too that it 'also takes variation in mood' – sometimes, he suggests, one needs to be relaxed or open to a particular emotion or to see the picture at a particular time of day. Literally and metaphorically, to appreciate a work fully we need to live with a picture and get to know it, to see it close up, move it about and so on (see Armstrong, 1996, pp. 142–143).

Fish and Coles (1998) offers an example of two people working together on producing a commentary. We found that this helped the process greatly. Since the critical commentary focuses on a piece of practice crystallized in a portrait, it is possible to share this with a critical friend whether or not they were privy to the original practice. In discussing the processes involved in preparing our commentary on our colleagues' practice we made the point that 'the basis of our own response to the writings . . . is a very careful reading, which attended to the writers' intentions as discernible from the writing, to the detail of meanings in each chapter and to how they are conveyed'. Indeed, we 'scrutinized each chapter in very considerable detail, seeking to understand what each writer is offering, seeking its themes and insights, looking at its elements, noting its form and structure as well as its focus and setting and its style and imagery'. We also said:

> we therefore read through the entire set of chapters, responding to them holistically, and then re-read them. We noted carefully during both readings what we believed the writers to be saying, making various checks against the text and sharing our perceptions of this. We came to all this open-mindedly. We also noted how the form and style underlined the content, by means of the shape and form of the piece, the judicious selection of vocabulary, the texture of language (style) and tone of voice. (Fish and Coles, 1998, p. 212)

We also reported that – once the overall impact of the pieces had been made – 'during our second reading we marked their text at any and all points where we noted something of significance' (Fish and Coles, 1998, p. 212).

In terms of where to begin, then, we made it clear that:

the discerned intentions of our writers then are proper starting and finishing points for a critical appreciation of their writing. In this case we mean their detailed as well as their overall intentions, some of which they themselves only discovered during the course of their writing. (Fish and Coles, 1998, p. 212)

But of course it is also important from the beginning that the critics reveal and consider their own interests, recognize and acknowledge their own subjectivities, values, assumptions and beliefs, and review their relationship (emotional as well as intellectual) with the portrait and the practice it takes as its subject. (It should be noted that this relationship may have changed over time.)

It is also important early in the proceedings to ensure that as full an understanding as possible of the context of the portrait and of its subject matter has been achieved in order that it can be properly seen and understood within its setting. If the quality and meaning of what has been achieved in a piece of practice is to be properly understood by both writer and readers, it is important to attend to the history and traditions which influence the practice. That is, a critical commentary needs to consider carefully the history of the practitioner and the present traditions of his or her profession, in order to discern and reveal the full significance of the particular piece of practice. This means providing enough information about the professional involved in the event (autobiographical information if the event is your own, biographical information provided by your subject if it is about someone else's practice), and enough detail about professional practice in general to enable the practice described to be properly understood as a particular example seen within the context of a more general way of working (representing either an example of it or a contrast to it).

Main activities

Eisner informs us that criticism proceeds not by pointing to the facts of the world but rather by intimation (Eisner, 1979, p. 201), and that criticism works by implication, innuendo, nuance, together with literal reference to the qualities of the work (Eisner, 1979, p. 203).

In attempting to 'discern the whispers of what lies just beyond [the portrait's] voiced details', we argued in Fish and Coles (1998, see p. 210) that this involves the following kinds of activity:

- pinpointing the writer's intentions and attitude to subject (which as well as being stated can be reached through imagery, tone, mood, style);
- getting beneath the surface of the words to the iceberg below;
- recognizing the themes and ideas being presented and explored and thinking about their significance and relating them to theoretical issues and to formal theory;
- highlighting the writers' sensibilities by drawing attention to nuance, mood and tone as well as imagery and style;
- considering how form and structure themselves convey, support and even elaborate upon content;
- looking at pattern and balance, continuity and development;
- considering the moral content as it emerges via style, tone and mood, and through the stated and the implied values, beliefs and assumptions;
- identifying and celebrating the spirit which shines through it.

Essentially this is achieved by picking out details, pointing to relationships, noting contrasts and counterpoint, in short, revealing the aesthetic order (see Armstrong, 1996, pp. 133–134). He points out that 'appreciation spirals outwards'. It also involves digging the values out of the figurative language, and looking at the basis of the description. But at the same time it has to be remembered that 'there is no value-free method of seeing' (Eisner, 1979, p. 105) and that we need always to 'consider the impact of our theories on our perceptions' (Eisner, 1979, p. 196). It also requires a systematic analysis and interpretation of the meanings that lie under the surface.

During this process we also have to be alert to our emotional responses to the portrait, and recognize them and the techniques which have evoked them, as well as responding at the emotional level to the original activities of the practice itself. The intellectual and the emotional responses are equally part of a critical commentary. As Armstrong says of art criticism:

> we have to feel and we have to be sensitive to colour and line, but we also have to understand the structure of the work, we have to

grasp the content and we have to evaluate intellectually the worth of certain contents. This is a process which involves bringing together just those qualities which, for the most part, daily life often keeps apart. Equally, we must not think that such rewarding experience could arise automatically as one stares hopefully at a picture. That just does not happen. (Armstrong, 1996, p. 141)

Further, the critic needs to keep a self-reflective eye upon his or her work. Again as Armstrong notes, 'The educated eye . . . knows when its associations and expectations are relevant and when they are not: it is not under the tyranny of the past, even though it is able, if need be, to draw upon the past; it has cultivated visual curiosity and attentiveness' (Armstrong, 1996, p. 115).

When the critic has uncovered and responded to all this, there will be a need to consider the portrait and the practice it has crystallized as a particular example of the more general work of that profession, and through this to consider the vision of practice enshrined in the portrait in relation to new ways of seeing and working in that profession. Only then will the significance of the understandings achieved become clear. Only then will those understandings be related to future possibilities.

But, of course, all this will lack credibility without recourse to the procedures through which the work is rendered reliable and valid. As was made clear in Chapter 5, these are not the same as those used in scientific or even social science research.

Ensuring reliability and validity, and justifying our judgements

What, then, needs to be attended to in order to assure readers that the investigations involved, and the commentary provided is rigorous and scholarly? Investigation in the Arts accepts and embraces subjectivity, and therefore questions about objectivity are irrelevant in this context. But rigour is always important. Again, it is achieved in different ways in the artistic/holistic paradigm as compared to the science and social science paradigms. Here, in working over the drafts, and in the detailed reference to the portrait in the commentary, care in the use of artistic and critical processes ensures rigour and promotes accuracy of detail *and spirit*. (Statements which strive for cold fact often fail to capture that deeper truth – truth to the spirit of the matter.) All this is also true of the various points at which reference is made to the wider world of professional theory and practice. The shiver of recognition by the reader is a strong indication that this work has the authority of realism. It is also credible where – and only where – a critical and questioning attitude (as indicated by the term critical commentary) balances the responsive and celebratory approach to achievements. It will be acceptable as properly scholarly where the critic's professional judgement ensures that the portrait as a whole and the practice to which it refers are appropriate and worthwhile subjects upon which professionals might focus a detailed investigation.

Further, the open recognition and declaration of the critic's values and beliefs, combined with the checking back to text (what Eisner calls referential adequacy) and rechecking authorial meaning, all indicate a concern for fairness and for providing the reader with all the evidence necessary to reconsider the case being put. (Though of course checking authorial meaning does not preclude the critic revealing new ways of reading the text.) For example, in Fish and Coles (1998) we said:

> it will be noted from this that we seek to avoid the abuse of criticism so often evident when the critic tries to make of or impose upon his or her subject, those meanings, intentions and concerns for which there is no evidence. We seek to respond to what the writers are seeking to say. Although what we offer is still our interpretation, we have tried to ensure that it responds to what is in the writing, by referencing our comments back to the original text, thus leaving the reader to decide ultimately on the value of our comments. We have also taken the precaution of sharing and checking out our responses with our writers. (Fish and Coles, 1998, p. 211)

The commentary is validated, then, by structural corroboration. This is:

> . . . process of [establishing] links that eventually create a whole that is supported by the bits of evidence that constitute it. Evidence is structurally corroborative when pieces of evidence validate each other, the story holds up, the pieces fit, it makes sense. (Eisner, 1979, p. 215)

The provision of carefully presented arguments and of clear supporting evidence drawn from the picture also allows the audience to examine the artist/writer's judgements and to consider critically those judgements made by the critic.

Evaluative judgements are endemic to critical commentaries, and Armstrong provides a striking image for the process of justifying our judgements as writers of critical commentaries. Recognizing that justifying our judgements (about art) comes in lots of small points, he argues that evaluative judgement emerges as critics become at home in the network of practices and traditions which they are studying and as these come to make more and more sense. He says:

> there does not emerge a single, primitive, basis for preference, rather lots and lots of little points are made, and this goes hand in hand with the development of a more discriminating and informed palate: none of which, perhaps, is decisive on its own, but cumulatively they approach justification. (Armstrong, 1996, p. 151)

He calls this Venetian Justification, saying that there is:

> no solid ground upon which the city is built. But by way of millions of piers driven into lagoon it does actually (still) stand, although no pier on its own can be thought of as uniquely supporting it. Our judgements of taste are like Venice: ultimately precarious, but nevertheless raising themselves beautifully above the water; there is no bedrock of justification to which they are attached, but the multiplicity of little supports allows us to approach security. (Armstrong, 1996, p. 151)

He also points out that, on this model, a poor judgement is one that is supported by very few, or flimsy, piers.

He also examines in detail the arguments about the intersubjective validity of judgements (which the practice of appreciation assumes). The argument concerns the notion that if a work sustains the judgement that it is of high artistic merit, on similar grounds, across a wide range of judges, then this gives ground for thinking that the judgement is intersubjectively valid, and that those who disagree with it have flawed judgement with respect to that work (Armstrong, 1996, p. 154). He comes to the conclusion that this idea is unprovable but is plausible (see Armstrong, 1996, p. 161).

Conclusion: new beginnings

These, then, are some of the activities and procedures involved in presenting a critical commentary. And with the production and sharing of that commentary, this small part of professional research and development will come to an end – except of course that the enlightenment it brings continues to affect our thinking and actions almost indefinitely. Indeed, the re-education of our perception and the extending of our vision is more like a beginning than an end, and is certainly likely to encourage professionals who engage in it to carry out further work of this kind.

But the only way of knowing this to be true is to try it. Do not be daunted by the length of the explanations in this book. It always takes longer to explain something than to do it. If necessary, re-read Part Three, and then have a go!

References

Adamson, B., Sinclair-Legge, G., Cusick, A. and Nordholm, L. (1994) Attitudes, values and orientation to professional practice: a study of Australian occupational therapists. *British Journal of Occupational Therapy*, 57, 476–480.

Agan, R. D. (1987) Intuitive knowing as a dimension of nursing. *Advances in Nursing Science*, 10, 63–70.

Armstrong, J. (1996) *Looking at Pictures: An Introduction to the Appreciation of Art*. Duckworth.

Auden, W. H. (1968) *Shorter Collected Poems, 1927–1957*. Faber.

Barthes, R. (1977) The death of the author. In *Image Music Text* (trans. Stephen Heath). Fontana, pp. 45–67.

Barton, A. (1971) Shakespeare: his tragedies. In *English Drama to 1710* (C. Ricks, ed.), The Sphere History of Literature in the English Language, Volume 3. Sphere Books, pp. 215–252.

Beckett, D. (1996) Critical judgement and professional practice. *Educational Theory*, 46, 135–149.

Beckingham, C. (1986) How the study of literature develops perceptive, sensitive nurses. *Australian Journal of Advanced Nursing*, 3, 15–20.

Beeston, S. and Simons, H. (1996) Physiotherapy practice: practitioners' perspectives. *Physiotherapy Theory and Practice*, 12, 231–242.

Benett, I. J. and Danczak, A. F. (1994) Terminal care: improving teamwork in primary care using significant event analysis. *European Journal of Cancer Care*, 3, 54–57.

Benner, P. (1984) *From Novice to Expert: Excellence and Power in Clinical Nursing Practice*. Addison-Wesley.

Benner, P. and Tanner, C. (1987) Clinical judgement: how expert nurses use intuition. *American Journal of Nursing*, January, pp. 23–31.

Benner, P. and Wrubel, J. (1982) Skilled clinical knowledge, the value of perceptual awareness. *Nurse Educator*, May–June, pp. 11–17.

Bennett, A. and Royle, N. (1995) *An Introduction to Literature, Criticism and Theory: Key Critical Concepts*. Prentice Hall–Harvester Wheatsheaf.

Berwick, D. M. (1996) A primer on leading the improvement of systems. *British Medical Journal*, 312, 619–622.

Bradley, C. P. (1992) Turning anecdotes into data – the critical incident technique. *Family Practitioner: an International Journal*, 9, 98–103.

Breunig, K. (1994) The art of painting meets the art of nursing. In *Art and Aesthetics in Nursing* (P. L. Chinn and M. J. Watson, eds). National League for Nursing Press, pp. 191–201.

Brigley, S., Young, Y., Littlejohns, P. and McEwen, J. (1996) Continuing education for medical professionals: a reflective model. *Postgraduate Medical Journal*, 73, 23–26.

Bullock, A. (1990) A case for the humanities: the Edward Boyle Memorial Lecture. *Royal Society of Arts Journal*, 138, 664–674.

Capra, F. (1983) *The Turning Point*. Flamingo.

Carper, B. A. (1978) Fundamental patterns of knowing in nursing. *Advances in Nursing Science*, 1, 13–23.

Carr, D. (1995) Is understanding the professional knowledge of teachers a theory–practice problem? *Journal of Philosophy of Education*, 29, 311–332.

Carr, W. (1995) *For Education: Towards Critical Educational Inquiry*. Open University Press.

Cervero, R. M. (1992) Professional practice, learning and continuing education: an integrated perspective. *International Journal of Lifelong Education*, 11, 91–101.

Chinn, P. L. (1994) Esthetics and the art of nursing. *Advances in Nursing Science*, 17, viii.

Chinn, P. L. and Kramer, M. K. (1995) *Theory and Nursing: a Systematic Approach*. Mosby Year Book Inc.

Chinn, P. L. and Watson, M. J. (eds) (1994) *Art and Aesthetics in Nursing*. National League for Nursing Press.

Coles, C. (1996) Undergraduate education and palliative care. *Palliative Medicine*, 10, 93–98.

Connelly, F. M. and Clandinin, D. J. (1986) On narrative method, personal philosophy and narrative units in the story of teaching. *Journal of Research in Science Thinking*, 23, 293–310.

Connelly, F. M. and Clandinin, D. J. (1990) Stories of experience and narrative inquiry. *Educational Research*, 19, 2–14.

Connelly, F. M. and Clandinin, D. J. (1995) Narrative and education. *Teachers and Teaching: Theory and Practice*, 1, 73–86.

Daiches, D. (1963) *Critical Approaches to Literature*. Longmans.

Davis, D. A., Thomson, M. A., Oxman, A. D. and Haynes, R. B. (1995) Changing physician performance: a systematic review of the effect of continuing medical education strategies. *Journal of the American Medical Association*, 274, 700–705.

Dawes, R. M. (1988) You can't systematize human judgement: dyslexia. In *Professional Judgement: a Reader in Clinical Decision-making* (J. Dowie and A. Elstein, eds). Cambridge University Press, pp. 150–162.

Dawson, S. W. (1970) *Drama and the Dramatic* (The Critical Idiom Series). Methuen.

Dickson, E. J. (1996) East meets West in the operating theatre. *The Sunday Telegraph*, 2 November, p. A7.

Diers, D. (1990) The art and craft of nursing. *American Journal of Nursing*, **90**, 65–66.

Dowie, J. and Elstein, A. (eds) (1988) *Professional Judgement: a Reader in Clinical Decision-Making.* Cambridge University Press.

Eddy, D. M. and Clanton, D. (1988) The art of diagnosis. In *Professional Judgement: a reader in clinical decision-making* (J. Dowie and A. Elstein, eds). Cambridge University Press, pp. 190–208.

Egan, K. (1988) *Teaching as Story Telling: An Alternative Approach to Teaching and Curriculum in the Elementary School.* Althouse Press.

Eisner, E. (1979) *The Educational Imagination: On the Design and Evaluation of School Programs.* Macmillan.

Eisner, E. (1983) The art and craft of teaching. *Educational Leadership*, **40**, 4–13.

Eisner, E. (1985) *The Art of Educational Evaluation: A Personal View.* Falmer Press.

Eisner, E. (1993) Forms of understanding and the future of educational research. *Educational Researcher*, **22**, 5–11.

Eisner, E. (1995) What artistically crafted research can help us understand about schools. *Educational Theory*, **45**, 1–6.

Eliot, T. S. (1963) *Collected Poems 1909–1962.* Faber & Faber.

Emerson, R. W. (1982) *Selected Essays.* Penguin Books.

Eraut, M. (1994) *Developing Professional Knowledge and Competence.* Falmer Press.

Eraut, M. (1995) Schön Shock: a case for reframing reflection-in-action? *Teachers and Teaching: Theory and Practice*, **1**, 9–23.

Fish, D. (1989) *Learning Through Practice in Initial Teacher Training: A Challenge for the Partners.* Kogan Page.

Fish, D. (1995a) *Quality Mentoring for Student Teachers: A Principled Approach to Practice.* David Fulton.

Fish, D. (ed.) (1995b) *Quality Learning for Student Teachers: University Tutors' Educational Practices.* David Fulton.

Fish, D. and Coles, C. (eds) (1998) *Developing Professional Judgement in Health Care: Learning through the Critical Appreciation of Practice.* Butterworth-Heinemann.

Fish, D. and Purr, B. (1991) *An Evaluation of Practice-based Learning in Continuing Education in Nursing, Midwifery and Health Visiting.* The English National Board for Nursing, Midwifery and Health Visiting.

Fish, D. and Twinn, S. (1997) *Quality Clinical Supervision in the Health Care Professions: Principled Approaches to Practice.* Butterworth-Heinemann.

Fish, D., Twinn, S. and Purr, B. (1990) *How to Enable Learning Through Professional Practice.* West London Press.

Ford, P. and Walsh, M. (1994) *New Rituals for Old: Nursing Through the Looking-glass.* Butterworth-Heinemann.

Freidson, E. (1994) *Professionalism Reborn: Theory, Prophesy and Policy.* Polity Press.

Gadamer, H. (1989) *Truth and Method*, 2nd rev. edn (trans. J. Weinscheimer and D. Marshall). Sheed and Ward.

Gilroy, P. (1993) Reflections on Schön: an epistemological critique and a practical alternative. *International Analysis of Teacher Education: Journal of Education for Teaching*, **19**, 83–89.

Ginger, J. (ed.) (1970) *An Approach to Criticism.* University of London Press.

Golby, M. (1981) Practice and theory. In *Rethinking Curriculum Studies* (M. Lawn and L. Barton, eds). Croom Helm, pp. 214–236.

Golby, M. (1993) *Case Study as Educational Research.* Fair Way Publications.

Golby, M. and Appleby, R. (1995) Reflective practice through critical friendship: some possibilities. *Cambridge Journal of Education*, **25**, 149–160.

Gore, J. M. (1991) Practicing what we preach: action-research and the supervision of student teachers. In *Issues and Practices in Inquiry-Oriented Teacher Education* (B. R. Tabachnick and K. M. Zeichner, eds). The Falmer Press, pp. 253–272.

Grahame-Smith, D. (1995) Evidence-based medicine: Socratic dissent. *British Medical Journal*, **310**, 1126–1127.

Gray, G. and Pratt, R. (eds) (1991) *Towards a Discipline of Nursing.* Churchill Livingstone.

Groundwater-Smith, S. (1984) The portrayal of schooling and the literature of fact. *Curriculum Perspectives*, **4**, 1–6.

Gudmundsdotter, S. (1991) Story maker, story teller. *Journal of Curriculum Studies*, **23**, 207–218.

Hagadorn, R. (1995) The Casson Memorial Lecture 1995: An emergent profession – a personal perspective. *British Journal of Occupational Therapy*, **58**, 324–331.

Hagadorn, R. (1997) Occupational therapy – a balancing act. *Conference Proceedings: Making a Difference* (19th National Conference of the Australian Association of Occupational Therapists). Promaco Conventions for the Association of Australian Occupational Therapists.

Hagar, P. (1997) Asking the right questions about professional practice: David Carr and beyond. In *Papers of the Philosophy of Education Society of Great Britain* – 4–6 April 1997. Philosophy of Education Society of Great Britain, pp. 112–118.

Haines, A. and Jones, R. (1994) Implementing findings of research. *British Medical Journal*, **308**, 1488–1492.

Hamilton, D., Jenkins, D., King, C. *et al.* (eds) (1977) *Beyond the Numbers Game.* Macmillan Education.

Hampton, D. (1994) Expertise: the true essence of nursing art. *Advances in Nursing Science*, **17**, 15–24.

Heath, I. (1995) *The Mystery of General Practice* (The John Fry Trust Fellowship). The Nuffield Provincial Hospitals Trust.

Higgs, J. and Jones, M. (eds) (1995) *Clinical Reasoning in Health Professions*. Butterworth-Heinemann.

Hildick, W. (1968) *Thirteen Types of Narrative*. Macmillan.

Holmes, C. (1991) Theory: where are we going and what have we missed along the way? In *Towards a Discipline of Nursing* (G. Gray, and R. Pratt, eds). Churchill Livingstone, pp. 435–460.

Holmes, J. (1996) Can poetry help us to become better psychiatrists? *Psychiatric Bulletin*, 20, 722–725.

Holt, M. (1996) The making of *Casablanca* and the making of curriculum. *Journal of Curriculum Studies*, 28, 241–251.

Hopkins, A. and Solomon, J. (1996) Can contracts drive clinical care? *British Medical Journal*, 313, 477–478.

Hoyle, E. (1974) Professionality, professionalism and the control of teaching. *London Educational Review*, 3, 13–18.

Hoyle, E. and John, P. (1995) *Professional Knowledge and Professional Practice*. Cassell.

Hunt, G. (1997) The human condition of the professional: discretion and accountability. *Nursing Ethics*, 4, 519–526.

Jacob, G. (ed.) (1951) *Tschaikovsky: Fantasy-Overture Romeo and Juliet*. The Penguin Scores Number 11.

Jalongo, M. R. (1992) Teachers' stories: our ways of knowing. *Educational Leadership*, 49, 68–79.

Johnson, J. (1994) A dialectical examination of nursing art. *Advances in Nursing Science*, 17, 1–14.

Joyce, J. (1965 [1914]) *The Dubliners*. Jonathan Cape.

Joyce, J. (1967 [1916]) *A Portrait of the Artist as a Young Man*. Jonathan Cape.

Katz, J. (1988) Why doctors don't disclose uncertainty. In *Professional Judgement: a Reader in Clinical Decision-making* (J. Dowie and A. Elstein, eds). Cambridge University Press, pp. 544–565.

Keen, T. and Shannon, A. (1991) Fish are the last to discover water. *Senior Nurse*, 11, 36–38.

Kemmis, S. (1995) Prologue: theorizing educational practice. In *For Education: Towards Critical Educational Inquiry* (W. Carr). Open University Press, pp. 1–18.

Kenner, H. (1955) *The Portrait* in perspective. In *James Joyce: Dubliners and A Portrait of the Artist as A Young Man: A Selection of Critical Essays* (Case Book Series) (M. Beja, ed.). Macmillan, pp. 124–150.

Kent, S. (1995) *Composition* (Eyewitness Art Series). Dorling Kindersley.

Kielhofner, G. (ed.) (1995) *A Model of Human Occupation: Theory and Application*, 2nd edn. Williams and Wilkins.

Landgrebe, B. and Winter, R. (1994) 'Reflective' writing in practice: professional support for the dying? *Educational Action Research*, 2, 83–94.

Langford, G. (1978) *Teaching as a Profession: an Essay in the Philosophy of Education*. Manchester University Press.

Langford, G. (1985) *Education Persons and Society: a Philosophical Enquiry*. Macmillan.

Larousse Encyclopedia of Mythology (1972) (New edition, fourth impression, trans. by R. Aidington and D. Ames.) Hamlyn.

Le Fanu, J. (1996) What cure for lack of respect? *The Sunday Telegraph*, 3 November, p. 4.

MacDonald, B. and Walker, R. (1977) Case study and the social philosophy of educational research. In *Beyond the Numbers Game – a Reader in Educational Evaluation* (D. Hamilton, D. Jenkins, C. King et al., eds). Macmillan Education, pp. 181–189.

McMahon, M. (1997) We have ways of making you teach. *The Sunday Telegraph*, 9 February, p. 32.

Maeve, M. K. (1994) Coming to moral consciousness through the art of nursing narratives. In *Art and Aesthetics in Nursing* (P. L. Chinn and M. J. Watson, eds). National League for Nursing Press, pp. 67–89.

Mattingly, C. and Fleming, M. (1994) *Clinical Reasoning: Forms of Inquiry in a Therapeutic Practice*. F. A. Davis Co.

Mole, P. (1992) *Acupuncture: Energy Balancing for Body, Mind and Spirit* (Health Essentials Series). Element.

Munby, H. (1986) Metaphor in the thinking of teachers: an exploratory study. *Journal of Curriculum Studies*, **18**, 197–209.

Oakeshott, M. (1962) The activity of being an historian. In *Rationalism in Politics and Other Essays*. Methuen, pp. 137–167.

Passmore, J. (1980) *The Philosophy of Teaching*. Duckworth Press.

Peterat, L. and Smith, G. (1996) Metaphoric reflections on collaboration in a teacher education practicum. *Educational Action Research*, **4**, 15–28.

Phenix, P. (1964) *Realms of Meaning: Philosophy of the Curriculum for General Education*. McGraw-Hill.

Piper, D. (1981) An introduction to painting and sculpture. In *Understanding Art: Appreciation, Method and Technique* (The Mitchell Beazley Library of Art). Mitchell Beazley, pp. 1–20.

Pringle, M., Bradley, C., Carmichael, C. et al. (1995) *Significant Event Auditing: A Study of the Feasibility and Potential of Case-Based Auditing in Primary Medical Care*. The Royal College of General Practitioners (Occasional Paper No. 70).

Proudfoot, R. (1971) Shakespeare: his career and development. In *English Drama to 1710* (C. Ricks, ed.), The Sphere History of Literature in the English Language, Volume 3. Sphere Books, pp. 148–165.

Radwany, S. M. and Adelson, B. H. (1987) The use of literary classics in teaching medical ethics to physicians. *Journal of the American Medical Association*, **257**, 1629–1631.

Ranson, R. (1994) *Distilling the Scene*. David and Charles.

Reed, J. and Procter, S. (eds) (1995) *Practitioner Research in Health Care: the Inside Story*. Chapman and Hall.

Rew, L. (1990) Intuition: nursing knowledge and the spiritual dimension of persons. *Holistic Nursing Practice*, **3**, 56–68.

Richardson, J. (1997) *Looking at Pictures: an Introduction to Art for Young People Through the Collection of the National Gallery*. A. and C. Black in association with National Gallery Publications.

Robb, A. and Murray, R. (1992) Medical humanities in nursing: thought provoking? *Journal of Advanced Nursing*, **17**, 1182–1187.

Roberts, C., Lewis, P., Crosby, D. *et al.* (1996) Prove it. *Health Service Journal*, 7 March, pp. 32–33.

Roberts, C., Colin-Thomé, D., Crosby, D. *et al.* (1996) The proof of the pudding . . . *Health Service Journal*, 14 March, p. 27.

Rogers, J. C. (1983) Eleanor Clarke Slagle Lectureship – clinical reasoning: the ethics, science, and art. *The American Journal of Occupational Therapy*, **37**, 601–616.

Rowland, G., Rowland, S. and Winter, R. (1990) Writing fiction as inquiry into professional practice. *Journal of Curriculum Studies*, **22**, 291–293.

Rudduck, J. and Hopkins, D. (eds) (1985) *Research as a Basis for Teaching: Readings from the Work of Lawrence Stenhouse.* Heinemann Educational.

Russell, T. and Munby, H. (1991) Reframing: the role of experience in developing teachers' professional knowledge. In *The Reflective Turn: Case Studies In and On Educational Practice* (D. Schön, ed.). The Teachers College Press, pp. 164–187.

Ruthven, K. K. (1969) *The Conceit* (The Critical Idiom Series). Methuen.

Schechner, R. and Appel, W. (eds) (1990) *By Means of Performance: Intercultural Studies of Theatre and Ritual.* Cambridge University Press.

Schön, D. A. (1983) *The Reflective Practitioner.* Basic Books.

Schön, D. A. (1987a) *Educating the Reflective Practitioner.* Jossey-Bass.

Schön, D. A. (1987b) Changing patterns in inquiry in work and living. *Journal of the Royal Society of Art Proceedings*, **135**, 225–231.

Schostak, J. F. (1985) Creating the narrative case record. *Curriculum Perspectives*, **5**, 7–13.

Shannon, A. (1987) A nursing opportunity. *Senior Nurse*, **7**, 10–15.

Sim, T. (1990) The concept of health. *Physiotherapy*, **76**, 423–428.

Sloboda, J. (1985) *The Musical Mind – the Cognitive Psychology of Music.* Oxford University Press.

Southgate, M. (1997) *One Hundred Covers and Essays from the Journal of the American Medical Association.* Mosby for the American Medical Association.

Spouse, J. (1994) Interviewing and the use of visual metaphors in social research. *British Educational Research Association Conference*, 8–11 September, 1994.

Stechow, W. (1990) *Pieter Bruegel the Elder.* Thames and Hudson.

Stenhouse, L. (1975) *An Introduction to Curriculum Research and Development.* Heinemann.

Stenhouse, L. (1980) Artistry and teaching: the teacher as the focus of research and development. In *Alternative Perspectives on School Improvement* (D. Hopkins and M. Wideen, eds). Falmer Press, pp. 90–101.

Strawson, P. F. (1974) *Freedom and Resentment.* Methuen.

Thow, M. and Murray, R. (1991) Medical humanities in physiotherapy: education and practice. *Physiotherapy*, **77**, 733–736.

Tooley, S. (1910) *The Life of Florence Nightingale.* Cassell.

Tripp, D. (1993) *Critical Incidents in Teaching: Developing Professional Judgement.* Routledge.

Vezeau, T. M. (1994a) Narrative inquiry in nursing. In *Art and Aesthetics in Nursing* (P. L. Chinn, and M. J. Watson, eds). National League for Nursing Press, pp. 41–66.

Vezeau, T. M. (1994b) Narrative in nursing practice and education. In *Art and Aesthetics in Nursing* (P. L. Chinn, and M. J. Watson, eds). National League for Nursing Press, pp. 161–190.

Vyvyan, J. (1968) *Shakespeare and the Rose of Love: a Study of the Early Plays in Relation to the Mediaeval Philosophy of Love.* Chatto and Windus.

Watson, J. (1985) *Nursing: the Philosophy and Science of Caring.* Colorado Associated University Press.

Watson, J. and Chinn, P. (1994) Introduction: art and aesthetic as passage between centuries. In *Art and Aesthetics in Nursing* (P. L. Chinn, and M. J. Watson, eds). National League for Nursing Press, pp. xiii–xvii.

Weber, S. (1993) The narrative anecdote in teacher education. *Journal of Education for Teaching,* 19, 71–82.

White, S. (1997) Evidence-based practice and nursing, the new panacea? *British Journal of Nursing,* 6, 175–178.

Winter, R. (1986) Fictional–Critical Writing. *Cambridge Journal of Education,* 3, 175–182.

Winter, R. (1988) Fictional–critical writing: an approach to case study research by practitioners and for in-service and pre-service work with teachers. In *The Enquiring Teacher: Supporting and Sustaining Teacher Research* (J. Nias and S. Groundwater-Smith, eds). Falmer Press, pp. 231–248.

Young-Mason, J. (1988) Literature as a mirror to compassion. *Journal of Professional Nursing,* 4, 299–301.

Index

264   Index